PRESCRIBING IN PREGNANCY

PRESCRIBING IN PREGNANCY

Edited by

PETER C RUBIN, DM, MRCP

*Wellcome Trust senior fellow, University
Department of Materia Medica, Stobhill
General Hospital, Glasgow*

Articles from the *British Medical Journal*
Published by the British Medical Journal
Tavistock Square, London WC1H 9JR

ISBN 0 7279 0174 5

Filmset and printed in Great Britain by
Latimer Trend & Company Ltd, Plymouth

Contents

General principles

PETER C RUBIN

Understanding of the multifaceted issues concerned in the use of drugs during pregnancy has lagged far behind the development of knowledge in other areas of therapeutics. This is partly because "thalidomide's long shadow" has slowed research that entails giving a drug to a pregnant woman.[1] A further reason is undoubtedly the difficulties (often more imagined than real) in performing interdisciplinary research. None the less, progress is being made, and several monographs on the clinical pharmacology of pregnancy have recently been published.[2-6]

This book is aimed at practising clinicians who prescribe drugs for women who are, or who may become, pregnant. The emphasis is on the clinically relevant aspects of research performed over the past 10 years or so. There are two introductory chapters: one on clinical pharmacology relevant to human pregnancy and the other on identifying fetal abnormality. The remaining chapters cover treatment during pregnancy of: minor ailments, bacterial infections, asthma, thromboembolic disease, psychiatric disorders, rheumatoid arthritis, cardiovascular disorders, endocrine diseases, and epilepsy.

Epidemiology of drug use during pregnancy

About 35% of women in the United Kingdom take drugs at least once during pregnancy, although only 6% take a drug during the first trimester.[7] This excludes iron and vitamin supplements and drugs used during delivery. The most commonly used drugs are non-narcotic analgesics, which are taken by 12·9% of women, antibacterial agents, taken by 10·3% of women, and antacids, taken by 7·4% of women. A recent study in The Netherlands produced similar findings: analgesics were taken by 12·3% of women, antibacterial agents by 11·6%, and antacids by 7·7%. Drugs such as anticonvulsants and bronchodilators, for which careful monitoring of dose is necessary, are each prescribed in about 1% of pregnancies.

Drug use during pregnancy has decreased considerably since the last major survey in the United Kingdom in the mid-1960s. Total use has fallen from just under 80% to 35%, while the percentage of women taking self administered drugs has fallen from 64% to 9%.[7] This may be due largely to the continued attention paid by the news media to drug induced fetal abnormality.[8]

In the puerperium the use of drugs increases substantially.[9] [10] One study showed that more than 99% of women received at least one drug, often an analgesic, during the first week after delivery.[9] This study also found that hypnotics were used by 36% of women in the puerperium. There was no difference in the pattern of prescribing between mothers who were breast feeding and those who were bottle feeding.

Effect of pregnancy on dose requirements

The physiological changes of pregnancy can lead to clinically important reductions in the blood concentrations of certain drugs.

Total body water increases by as much as 8 litres during pregnancy,[11] [12] which provides a substantially increased volume within which drugs can be distributed.

Serum proteins relevant to drug binding undergo considerable changes in concentration.[13] Albumin, which binds acidic drugs such as phenytoin, decreases in concentration by up to 10 g/l.[14] The main implication of this change is in the interpretation of drug concentrations, which is discussed below.

Liver metabolism increases during pregnancy,[15] but liver blood flow does not.[16] Drugs with a rate of elimination which depends on the activity of liver enzymes can show large increases in clearance during pregnancy. Phenytoin is cleared at twice the rate found in non-pregnant women,[17] and theophylline undergoes similar changes (figure). In contrast, drugs which are eliminated at a rate mainly dependent on liver blood flow, such as propranolol, show no change in clearance during pregnancy.[18]

Renal plasma flow has almost doubled by the last trimester of pregnancy.[19] Drugs which are eliminated unchanged by the kidney

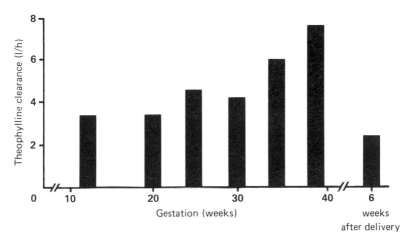

Theophylline clearance calculated from steady state concentrations in a pregnant woman with asthma. Having been controlled before pregnancy on 250 mg every 12 hours, by the end of pregnancy this patient had subtherapeutic concentrations despite receiving 1500 mg/day.

are usually eliminated more rapidly, but so far this has been shown to be clinically important in only a few cases. For example, ampicillin clearance doubles during pregnancy[20] and the dose used for systemic infections should be doubled. In urinary infections no change in dose is necessary.

The major consequence of these physiological changes is that some drugs—notably, anticonvulsants and theophylline derivatives—can undergo changes in distribution and elimination which lead to ineffective treatment because of inadequate drug concentrations in the blood.

Therapeutic drug monitoring during pregnancy

Among the drugs for which plasma concentrations would normally be measured those most likely to be encountered during pregnancy are anticonvulsants and theophylline derivatives. Because important changes in concentration may occur drug concentrations should be measured at monthly intervals throughout pregnancy and again one week and four weeks after delivery. The dose required usually increases as gestation progresses, particularly in the third trimester, and decreases in the puerperium. The increase may be large—for example, a patient who is normally well controlled taking 300 mg of phenytoin a day may require 600 mg a day by the end of pregnancy just to stay at the bottom of the therapeutic range.

Two points should be considered when interpreting drug concentrations during pregnancy.

Protein binding—The reduction in albumin concentration during pregnancy leads to a decrease in the measured concentrations of drugs which are highly bound, such as phenytoin. The increased amount of drug which is unbound will, however, be available for both distribution out of the blood and for elimination from the body. The net result of the change in albumin concentration on phenytoin is that the total level falls but the free level is virtually unchanged. Only the free (unbound) drug is pharmacologically active, and so if the laboratory gives drug concentrations as total drug the therapeutic range should be revised downwards. As a rule of thumb, the concentration of the drug should be kept at the bottom of the usual therapeutic range.

Therapeutic range—It is not clear whether pregnancy alters the effects of drugs. This is an important matter, but one which is difficult to study. Apart from the pharmacokinetic considerations detailed above, it is possible that established therapeutic ranges might be inappropriate during pregnancy because of changes in the relation between drug concentration and effect.

Passage of drugs to the fetus

Much of the published work on the transfer of drugs across the placenta is concerned with the rate of transfer, but except in the context of single doses—for example, at the time of delivery—this is not the major issue. The placenta is essentially a lipid barrier between the maternal and fetal circulations. Drugs cross the placenta by passive diffusion. A lipid soluble, un-ionised drug of low molecular weight will cross the placenta more rapidly than a more polar drug. Given time, however, most drugs will achieve roughly equal concentrations on each side of the placenta. For example, after a single dose of indomethacin the ratio of cord to maternal plasma concentration is 0·5:1 at two hours but 1:1 at five hours.[21] A similar example is provided by the β blockers. Researchers thought that a polar drug like atenolol might have limited transfer to the fetus, but on long term dosing this was found not to be the case.[22] Thus the practical view to take when prescribing drugs during pregnancy is that transfer of drugs to the fetus is inevitable. The only notable exception to this rule is heparin, which is so large and so polar that its transfer across the placenta is negligible.

Breast feeding

As with the transfer of drugs across the placenta, much has been written on the theoretical aspects of passage of drugs into breast milk, but the relevance of these publications is equally doubtful. Virtually all drugs cross into breast milk. Previous dilution in the mother's body, however, coupled with the volume of milk consumed usually means that the dose administered to the baby is clinically unimportant.

There are three main categories of drugs so far as breast feeding is concerned.

(1) Drugs which are undetectable in the baby. These include warfarin, which is so highly bound to maternal proteins that it is undetectable even in breast milk,[23] and aminoglycosides, which are not absorbed from the gastrointestinal tract of normal infants.[24]

(2) Drugs which reach the baby but in an insignificant dose. These include most drugs used in everyday practice: non-narcotic analgesics,[25] non-steroidal anti-inflammatory drugs,[26] penicillin and cephalosporin antibiotics,[27] antihypertensive drugs,[28] bronchodilator inhalers, and anticonvulsants (with the exception of barbiturates).[29] Special mention should be made here of two drugs which often feature in consultation requests to this department. Firstly, oral contraceptives containing low doses of oestrogen do not suppress established lactation and are not harmful to the baby. Secondly, metronidazole appears to be safe for the baby but causes the milk to have a bitter taste, which may impair feeding.

(3) Drugs which reach the baby in sufficient dose to be harmful. These are listed in the table.

Commonly used drugs which are contraindicated in women who are breast feeding

Laxatives	Lithium
Amiodarone	Opiates
Ephedrine and pseudoephedrine	Carbimazole
Barbiturates	Iodine (propylthiouracil seems to be safe)
Benzodiazepines	Cytotoxics and immunosuppressant drugs
Bromide salts	

Conclusion

The use of drugs during pregnancy and in the puerperium requires that a fine balance should be maintained. No harm should be allowed to befall the baby because of the drug, but equally no harm must come to the mother or baby because a disease is being inadequately treated. The aim of this book is to provide the information on which a clinical decision can be made.

1 Anonymous. Thalidomide's long shadow [Editorial]. *Br Med J* 1976;ii:1155–6.
2 Lewis P. *Clinical pharmacology in obstetrics*. Bristol: Wright, 1983.
3 Krauer B, Krauer F, Hytton F. *Drug prescribing during pregnancy*. Edinburgh: Churchill Livingstone, 1984.
4 Kuemmerle HP, Brendel K. *Clinical pharmacology in pregnancy*. New York: Thieme-Stratton, 1983.
5 Eskes TKAB, Finster M. *Drug therapy during pregnancy*. London: Butterworths, 1985.
6 Stirrat GM, Beeley L. Prescribing in pregnancy. *Clinics in Obstetrics and Gynaecology* 1986;**13**:161–413.
7 Rubin PC, Craig GS, Gavin K, Sumner D. Prospective survey of use of therapeutic drugs, alcohol and cigarettes during pregnancy. *Br Med J* 1986;**292**:81–3.
8 Orme ML. The debendox saga. *Br Med J* 1985;**291**:918–9.
9 Passmore CM, McElnay JC, D'Arcy PF. Drugs taken by mothers in the puerperium: inpatient survey in Northern Ireland. *Br Med J* 1984;**289**:1593–6.
10 Lewis PJ, Boyland P, Bulpitt CJ. An audit of prescribing in obstetric service. *Br J Obstet Gynaecol* 1980;**87**:1043–5.
11 Hytten FE, Leitch I. *The physiology of pregnancy*. Oxford: Blackwell Scientific, 1971.
12 Pirani BBK, Campbell DM, McGillivray I. Plasma volume in normal first pregnancy. *Journal of Obstetrics and Gynaecology of the British Commonwealth* 1973;**80**:884–7.
13 Studd J. The plasma proteins in pregnancy. *Clinics in Obstetrics and Gynaecology* 1975;**2**:285–300.
14 Reboud P, Groulade J, Groslambert, P, Colomb, M. The influence of normal pregnancy and the postpartum state on plasma proteins in lipids. *Am J Obstet Gynecol* 1963;**86**:820–8.
15 Davis M, Simmons CJ, Dordoni B, Maxwell JO, Williams R. Induction of hepatic enzymes during normal human pregnancy. *Journal of Obstetrics and Gynaecology of the British Commonwealth* 1973;**80**:690–4.
16 Munnel EW, Taylor HC. Liver blood flow in pregnancy—hepatic vein catheterisation. *J Clin Invest* 1947;**26**:952–6.
17 Lander CM, Smith MT, Chalk JB, *et al*. Bioavailability in pharmacokinetics of phenytoin during pregnancy. *Eur J Clin Pharmacol* 1984;**27**:105–10.
18 O'Hare MF, Kinney CD, Murnaghan JA, McDevitt DG. Pharmacokinetics of propranolol during pregnancy. *Eur J Clin Pharmacol* 1984;**27**:583–7.

19 Dunlop W. Investigations into the influence of posture on renal plasma flow and glomerular filtration rate during late pregnancy. *Br J Obstet Gynaecol* 1976;**83**:17–23.
20 Philipson A. Pharmacokinetics of ampicillin during pregnancy. *J Infect Dis* 1977;**136**:370–6.
21 Traeger A, Noschel H, Zaumseil J. Zur pharmacokinetik von Indomethazin bei Schwangeren, Kreissenden une deren Neugeboronen. *Zentralb Gynakol* 1973;**95**:635–41.
22 Rubin PC, Butters L, Reynolds B, *et al.* Atenolol elimination in the neonate. *Br J Clin Pharmacol* 1983;**16**:659–62.
23 Orme ML, Lewis PJ, Serling MJ. Can mothers given warfarin breast feed their infants? *Br Med J* 1977;i:1564–5.
24 Milner RDG. Gentamicin in the newborn. *Postgrad Med J* 1974;**50**(suppl 7):40–4
25 Berlin CM, Pascuzzi MJ, Jaffe SJ. Excretion of salicylate in human milk. *J. Clin Pharmacol* 1980;**27**:245–6.
26 Needs, CJ, Brooks PM. Antirheumatic medication during lactation. *British Journal of Rheumatology* 1985;**24**:291–7.
27 Lipman AG. Antimicrobial agents in breast milk. *Modern Medicine* 1977;**45**:89–90.
28 Liedholm H, Melander A, Bitzan PO, *et al.* Accumulation of atenolol and metoprolol in human breast milk. *Eur J Clin Pharmacol* 1981;**20**:229–31.
29 Nau H, Cuhnz W, Egger HJ, Rating D, Helge H. Anticonvulsants during pregnancy and lactation. *Clin Pharmacokinet* 1982;**7**:508–43.

Identifying abnormalities

MARTIN J WHITTLE, KEVIN P HANRETTY

Drugs taken during pregnancy create concern whether they are self administered or medically prescribed. The number of mothers who take drugs during pregnancy is not known, but a survey in the United States showed that about 45% of women may use at least one drug on prescription, and many more use drugs bought over the counter.[1] A recent prospective study in the United Kingdom, however, suggested that only about 10% of women took drugs in early pregnancy.[2]

Defects occur in about 2% to 3% of babies at birth, of which about 25% are of genetic origin and 65% are of unknown aetiology. Only 2% to 3% of defects are thought to arise in association with drug treatment.[3] The effect of a particular drug on the developing fetus depends on several features, including the type of agent and the gestational age at which it was taken.

The aim of this article is to provide a guide for doctors treating

Teratogenic effects of drugs

Drug	Effect	Incidence	Prenatal diagnosis
Lithium	Cardiac defects (Ebstein's complex)	10–12%	Feasible
Warfarin	Chondrodysplasia punctata Facial anomalies	5%	Unlikely
	Severe anomalies of the central nervous system	4%	Feasible
Phenytoin	Craniofacial Limb Growth deficiencies	30%	Feasible
Primidone and phenobarbitone	Facial clefting Cardiac anomalies	Unknown	Feasible
Sodium valproate	Central nervous system	2–3%	Feasible
Sex hormones	Cardiac defects Multiple anomalies	Unknown	Feasible

pregnant women who have taken, or who are currently taking, drugs. Advice depends on the following: (a) knowledge of the timing of embryonic and fetal development because preparations taken outside the critical phase are unlikely to be teratogenic; (b) the precise nature of the drug so that the teratogenic effect may be determined (table); and (c) whether the teratogenic effect is likely to be sufficiently apparent to make prenatal diagnosis feasible.

Timing of embryonic and fetal development

Several important phases in human development are recognised (fig 1).

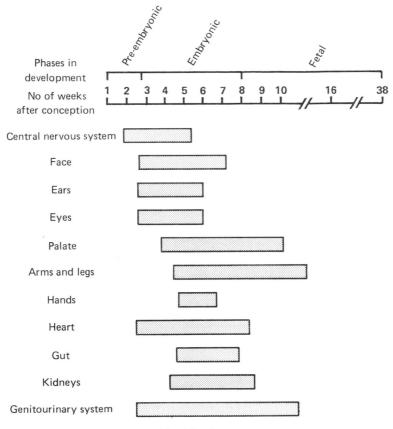

FIG 1—Timing of embryonic and fetal development.

During the pre-embryonic phase, from conception until 17 days, implantation, blastocyst formation, and gastrulation take place. During this time the result of an insult to the developing organism is either death and abortion (or resorption) or survival intact through multiplication of the still totipotential cells to replace those which have been lost.

Embryonic development, from 18 to 55 days after conception, is when the basic steps in organogenesis occur. This is the period of maximum sensitivity since not only are tissues differentiating rapidly but damage to them becomes irreparable. The earlier in this period the insult occurs the greater the likely effect.

During the fetal phase, from 56 days to term, the effects of drugs are usually limited to defects of growth and functional loss rather than gross structural abnormalities.

Drugs and their teratogenic effects

Extensive reviews on the teratogenic effects of drugs have recently been published.[4][5] The teratogenicity of some more commonly used drugs is briefly described here and covered more comprehensively in later chapters.

Antibiotics

Commonly used drugs, such as penicillins and cephalosporins, do not appear to be teratogenic.[5] In the case of antituberculous drugs ethambutol and isoniazid have a good safety record. Streptomycin causes deafness. Rifampicin, which causes neural tube defects and facial clefting in mice, is associated with a human fetal abnormality rate two to three times higher than ethambutol or isoniazid[6] and should be avoided if possible in the first trimester. Ethionamide has been associated with exomphalos and exencephaly and should also be avoided.

Psychotropic drugs

The benzodiazepines have been incriminated in the formation of oral clefts, though their teratogenicity has been disputed.[7] Tricyclic antidepressants and phenothiazines are not associated with fetal abnormality.[5]

10

Lithium, which is used in the treatment of affective disorders, is associated with an incidence of fetal abnormality of about 12%.[8] The cardiovascular system is more often affected with coarctation, patent ductus arteriosus, and mitral and tricuspid atresias being reported. The rare condition of Ebstein's anomaly, in which the tricuspid valve is distorted and displaced, occurred in a third of the affected babies and overall is about 500 times more common in the babies of women who take lithium.

Anticoagulants

Oral anticoagulants have been recognised as teratogens for several years[9] and are associated with three main types of abnormality.[10] Firstly, the abortion rate is increased by up to 50%. Secondly, anticoagulants can cause a well defined embryopathy, which includes bone stippling (chondrodysplasia punctata) and nasal hypoplasia. Both of these abnormalities occur more commonly, though not exclusively, with treatment during the first trimester. The overall incidence of the embryopathy is about 5%. Finally, there is a risk of serious abnormalities of the central nervous system, thought to result from dorsal midline dysplasia, which include absence of the corpus callosum, Dandy-Walker syndrome, and encephalocoeles.

Anticonvulsants

A twofold to fourfold increase in the incidence of malformations has been found among the babies of epileptic mothers. These include orofacial clefts and cardiac malformations (for example, septal defects), skeletal anomalies (talipes and hip dislocations), microcephaly, and neural tube defects.

The phenytoin syndrome, which occurs in up to 30% of exposed babies, comprises craniofacial abnormalities (depressed nasal ridge, hypertelorism, clefts), limb defects (hypoplasia of distal phalanges, digital thumb, hip dislocation), and intrauterine and postnatal growth deficiencies as well as neck and rib defects and umbilical hernias.[11,12]

Primidone and phenobarbitone may be teratogenic when combined with phenytoin,[13] though the evidence for their teratogenicity when used alone is not strong. Both have been associated with facial clefting and cardiac defects.

Sodium valproate, introduced as a useful alternative to other anticonvulsants, seems to be an important teratogen and is particularly likely to produce neural tube defects, with an incidence of about 2·5%.[14] It appears to cause spina bifida much more often than anencephaly the ratio being 5:1 with sodium valproate compared with a normal ratio of 1·25–2·25:1.

Carbamazepine does not appear to be teratogenic, although problems might arise when it is combined with other agents; it should therefore be used alone whenever possible.[13]

Immunosuppressive drugs

Pregnancy in women who have undergone renal transplantation and who are taking drugs such as azathioprine and prednisolone is becoming increasingly common. Studies on patients with ulcerative colitis and Crohn's disease, however, show little evidence that either agent is teratogenic in humans.[15]

Sex hormones

Hormone preparations taken in early pregnancy include the oral contraceptive pill and those used in threatened abortion and, unusually now, the hormone pregnancy test. Despite numerous studies, the teratogenic effects of hormones remain uncertain. Three main groups of abnormalities may occur: limb reductions; cardiac defects, especially transposition of the great vessels; and central nervous system defects such as hydrocephaly and neural tube lesions. The constellation of disorders termed VACTERAL (vertebral, anal atresia, cardiac, tracheo-oesophageal atresia, renal and limb defects) has been significantly associated with ingestion of hormones in early pregnancy in some studies.[16]

Management of pregnancy and potential teratogenesis

Teratogenesis concerns two main groups of patients: women already taking drugs for a chronic underlying illness and those who have taken a single course of treatment unaware of an early pregnancy. Undoubtedly, women in the former group should be counselled before their pregnancy so that they are fully aware of the risks of teratogenesis and how the risk of fetal malformation may be reduced. Such an approach demands close cooperation between physicians, general practitioners, and the prenatal diagnostic team. Regrettably, all too often the patient first presents in pregnancy. Under these circumstances we suggest the following scheme, which aims to establish accurately gestational age at the time of exposure to the drugs and the potential of prenatal diagnosis (fig 2).

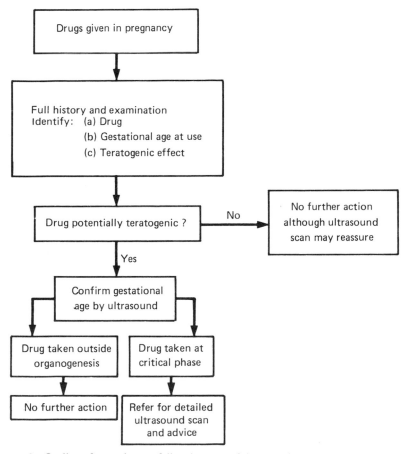

FIG 2—Outline of procedure to follow in cases of drug use in pregnancy.

History

Menstruation—A careful record of the recent dates of periods and the menstrual cycle should always be sought. Gestational age is more likely to be correct if the first day of the last period has been noted and the preceding cycles were regular (every 28 days), although even then up to 15% of calculations will be wrong by 14 days or more.[17]

Conception—It is always worth inquiring whether the woman knows when conception occurred; occasionally, remarkably accurate calculations are made.

Treatment—Once the gestational age has been established the exact time of exposure to the drugs must be determined. This may require a review of the patient's notes either from the general practitioner or the hospital. Careful identification of the drugs taken is vital, not just by the group—"I think it was something for my nerves"—but by name. The possibility that more than one drug was taken should also be considered. The patient may forget to mention the most important drug, and taking several drugs together may result in a higher incidence of teratogenesis. Patients should also be asked about self medication as they may report only medically prescribed preparations.

Investigation: establishing gestational age

Accurate estimation of gestational age is essential. Although a good history will help, dating by ultrasound scanning using fetal crown-rump length or, between 12 and 20 weeks, the biparietal diameter should allow the dates to be calculated to within about a week. With these data the exact stage in pregnancy at which treatment was given can be established. Quite often it can be shown that the mother was either not even pregnant at the time of exposure or had passed the time at which teratogenesis would be likely to occur.

Investigation: prenatal diagnosis

If drugs were taken at a critical gestational age the most effective method of excluding fetal anomaly is by high resolution ultrasound scanning. In optimal conditions this provides extraordinarily good images of the fetal brain and spine, the heart, the arms, legs, and hands, and the face (fig 3).

Fetal anomalies associated with teratogens may be broadly grouped into: defects of the central nervous system, cardiovascular system, and arms and legs; facial clefting; and multisystem defects. Most structural anomalies should be detectable by about 20 to 22 weeks, although this depends on several different factors, and it is not possible to provide exact rates of detection.

Central nervous system—One of the commonest indications for ultrasound examination in pregnancy is to exclude neural tube defects. Anencephaly can usually be identified about 12 weeks after the last period, but spina bifida is often more subtle and is best detected at 16 to 18 weeks. The predictive ability of ultrasound examination depends on good equipment, a high level of training, good fetal position, and a mother who is not excessively obese. In one series of neural tube defects all cases of anencaphaly were detected as well as 96 of 102 cases of spina bifida. In two cases spina bifida was wrongly diagnosed.[18]

The value of measuring maternal serum α fetoprotein concentration and performing amniocentesis is debatable in patients already referred for a detailed scan, when a lesion would be unlikely to be missed. If fetal views are poor, however, amniocentesis would be indicated in the presence of increased serum α fetoprotein concentrations. The high incidence of spina bifida in the babies of patients taking sodium valproate would certainly indicate the need for amniocentesis if views were unsatisfactory.[19]

Cardiovascular system—Fetal cardiology is a relatively recent development reflecting the vast improvements in the quality of imaging. Most serious heart defects, particularly those of connection, should be detectable by 16 to 18 weeks.[20] The basic requirement in cardiac scanning is to obtain a four chamber view, which, if normal, will exclude many important abnormalities. Gross defects, such as Ebstein's complex associated with lithium, have been detected by scan.[21]

Deformities of the arms and legs—Although it is relatively easy to measure the fetal limbs, abnormalities of growth may not become apparent until later in pregnancy.[22] Gross deformities of the type associated with thalidomide should, however, be detected by 16 weeks. Abnormalities of the hands and even equinus deformities of the feet may well be seen given optimal conditions.

15

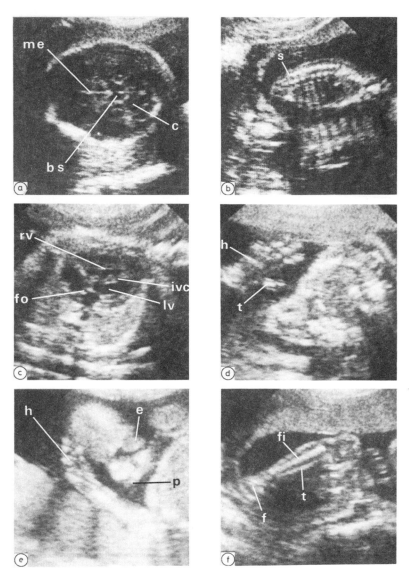

FIG 3—Ultrasound scans of (a) fetal brain (me = midline echo, bs = brain stem, c = cerebellum); (b) fetal spine (s); (c) fetal heart, showing the four chambers (rv = right ventricle, lv = left ventricle, ivs = intraventricular septum, fo = foramen ovale); (d) fetal hand (h = hand, t = thumb); (e) fetal face (e = eyelid, p = philtrum, h = hand); and (f) leg (t = tibia, fi = fibula, f = foot).

Facial clefting—This appears to be a common feature of teratogenesis, and, although not usually in itself an indication for terminating pregnancy, the display of normality may be some comfort to anxious parents. Fig 3e shows the clarity with which the fetal face can be seen.

Multiple anomalies—This group of anomalies can often be detected carly in pregnancy and usually by 16 weeks. In the VACTERAL complex features of the arms, legs, kidneys, and heart should be detectable by 18 to 20 weeks. Vertebral defects may be seen earlier, but tracheo-oesophageal fistula and anal atresia may not be diagnosed until delivery.

Conclusions

The exact role of drugs in producing fetal abnormalities remains uncertain, and some apparently unexplained fetal anomalies may be the result of a forgotten toxic insult. We hope that this chapter will be a useful guide to practitioners consulted about possible teratogenesis. In general terms we recommend the formation of a team, comprising a clinical pharmacologist and members of a prenatal diagnostic unit, which could provide rapid and effective advice.

1 Schardein JL. Current status of drugs as teratogens in man. *Prog Clin Biol Res* 1985;163C:147–53.
2 Rubin PC, Craig GF, Gavin K, Sumner D. Prospective survey of use of therapeutic drugs, alcohol and cigarettes during pregnancy. *Br Med J* 1986;292:81–3.
3 Wilson JG. Present status of drugs as teratogens in man. *Teratology* 1977;7:3–16.
4 Brendal K, Duhamel RC, Shephard TH. Embryotoxic drugs. *Int J Biol Res Pregnancy* 1985;6:1–54.
5 Greenberg G, Inman WHW, Weatherall JAC, Adelstein AN, Haskey JC. Maternal drug histories and congenital abnormalities. *Br Med J* 1977;ii:853–6.
6 Snieder DE, Layde PM, Johnson MW, Lyle MA. Treatment of tuberculosis during pregnancy. *Am Rev Resp Dis* 1980;122:65–79.
7 Weber LWD. Benzodiazepines in pregnancy-academic debate or teratogenic risk. *Int J Biol Res Pregnancy* 1985;6:151–67.
8 Linden S, Rich CL. The use of lithium during pregnancy and lactation. *J Clin Psychiatry* 1983;44:358–61.
9 Bloomfield DK. Fetal deaths and malformations associated with the use of coumarin derivatives in pregnancy. *Am J Obstet Gynecol* 1980;107:883–8.
10 Hall JG, Pauli RM, Wilson KA. Maternal and fetal sequelae of anticoagulation during pregnancy. *Am J Med* 1980;68:122–40.
11 Kelly TD. Teratogenicity of anticonvulsant drugs: review of the literature. *Am J Med Genet* 1984;19:413–34.
12 Albengres E, Tillement JP. Phenytoin in pregnancy: a review of the reported risks. *Int J Biol Res Pregnancy* 1983;4:71–4.
13 Brodie MJ. Epilepsy, anticonvulsants and pregnancy. In: Chadwick DW, Ross E, eds. *Epilepsy in young people*. Chichester: Wiley (in press).

14 Lindhout D, Schmidt D. In utero exposure to valproate and neural tube defect. *Lancet* 1986;i:1392–3.
15 Witter FR, King TM, Blake DA. The effects of chronic gastrointestinal medication on the fetus and neonate. *Obstet Gynecol* 1980;**58**:798–848.
16 Schardein JL. Congenital anomalies and hormones during pregnancy. A clinical review. *Teratology* 1980;**22**:251–70.
17 Persson PH, Kullander S. Long term experience of general ultrasound screening in pregnancy. *Am J Obstet Gynecol* 1982;**146**:942–7.
18 Campbell S, Smith P, Pearce JM. The ultrasound diagnosis of neural tube defects and other craniospinal abnormalities. In: Rodeck CH, Nicoliades KH, eds. Prenatal diagnosis. Proceedings of the 11th study group of the Royal College of Obstetricians and Gynaecologists. London: Royal College of Obstetricians and Gynaecologists, 1983:245–57.
19 Weinbaum PJ, Cassidy SB, Vintzileos AM, Campbell WA, Ciarleglio L, Nòchimson DJ. Prenatal detection of a neural tube defect after fetal exposure to valproic acid. *Obstet Gynecol* 1986;**67**:31–3.
20 Allan LD. Examining the fetal heart—commentary. *Br J Obstet Gynaecol* 1986;**93**:305–6.
21 Allan LD, Desai G, Tynan MJ. Prenatal echocardiographic screening for Ebstein's anomaly for mothers on lithium therapy. *Lancet* 1982;ii:875–6.
22 Connor JM, Connor RAC, Sweet EM, *et al*. Lethal neonatal chondrodysplasias in the West of Scotland 1970–83. *Am J Med Genet* 1985;**22**:243–53.

Treatment of common minor ailments

C W HOWDEN

A number of common minor disorders may occur in pregnancy and require drug treatment for control of symptoms. These include headache and musculoskeletal pains as well as a variety of gastrointestinal complaints, including heartburn, nausea, vomiting, dyspepsia, and constipation. This chapter reviews the drugs used to treat such complaints with respect to efficacy and safety and appraises the available evidence in an attempt to recommend the safest drugs.

Use of analgesics

Simple analgesics are the commonest drugs taken in pregnancy and are self administered. Aspirin, paracetamol, ibuprofen, and a variety of analgesic combinations are available in Britain without prescription. Many women consume analgesics in the early stages of pregnancy before realising they are pregnant. Collecting and interpreting controlled data on exposure to analgesics and the incidence of congenital defects are therefore difficult.

Aspirin

Evidence linking ingestion of aspirin to fetal malformations is suggestive but inconclusive. Massive doses of aspirin given to pregnant rats cause congenital skeletal and eye defects.[1] Many of the studies suggesting a teratogenic effect of aspirin in humans have been retrospective case-control studies. For example, among 833 women who had given birth to malformed babies there was a higher incidence of ingestion of aspirin during early pregnancy than in a control group.[2] In a large prospective cohort study of more than 50 000 women, however, no increase in congenital abnormalities was found in the babies of mothers who had taken aspirin during pregnancy when compared with control patients who had not taken aspirin.[3] Aspirin has been thought to cause a reduction in birth weight and an increase in the stillbirth rate.[4] In a prospective cohort study of more than 41 000 women, however, the stillbirth rate was 1·4% both in women who consumed large quantities of aspirin and those who took no aspirin during pregnancy.[5] Similarly, the neonatal death rate was 1·1% in both groups.

Aspirin is freely transferable across the placenta and is excreted by the newborn infant at a slower rate than in adults owing to immaturity of the excretory pathways.[6] The infant of a woman who ingested regular therapeutic doses of aspirin throughout pregnancy took five days to eliminate the drug.[6]

One potential problem of aspirin in newborn infants is its effect on haemostatic mechanisms. In a case-control study haemostasis was normal in 33 of 34 pairs of mothers and infants where there was no history of aspirin ingestion.[7] There were, however, abnormalities of platelet adhesiveness in most of the infants whose mothers had taken aspirin within five days of delivery. There was also a higher incidence of minor bleeding in the babies whose mothers had taken aspirin. Furthermore, intrapartum blood loss from the mothers was greater in those who had recently taken aspirin.

The possible teratogenic effect of aspirin, together with its well documented adverse effects on platelet function and haemostasis when taken in late pregnancy, suggest that aspirin should be avoided in pregnancy, particularly in the treatment of minor disorders. Non-steroidal anti-inflammatory drugs are discussed in the chapter on antirheumatic therapy (p 59).

Paracetamol

The effects of paracetamol during pregnancy have not been studied as extensively as those of aspirin, but it seems to be generally safe. Studies in animals have shown no adverse effects on fetal or placental growth.[8] Paracetamol does not have the same effect on clotting as aspirin and for this reason alone is preferable for use in pregnancy. There is nothing to suggest that paracetamol in normal dosage is associated with any specific problems during pregnancy or breast feeding, and it is recommended as the mild analgesic of choice.[9]

Treatment of nausea and vomiting

Although common in early pregnancy, nausea and vomiting are generally of short duration and can often be managed without drugs. Patients should be reassured and advised to take small frequent meals and to avoid large amounts of fluid. Drug treatment is often necessary, however, if symptoms are severe or prolonged. Antiemetic drugs have been linked to a number of congenital defects. One large prospective series showed an association between vomiting in early pregnancy and certain congenital abnormalities, but no correlation could be established with any specific antiemetic drug.[10] This led to the proposal that it was vomiting rather than antiemetic treatment which was causally associated with birth defects. In a prospective study of more than 16 000 women, however, there was no difference in the incidence of congenital defects between those who had vomited in pregnancy and those who had not.[11] The authors concluded that any increased risk in women taking antiemetic drugs was related to the drugs rather than the vomiting and that the risk was low in any case. Specific drugs are considered below.

Debendox

Debendox, a combination of dicyclomine, doxylamine, and pyridoxine, was highly successful in the management of nausea and vomiting during pregnancy. Sporadic case reports linking its use to congenital abnormalities caused concern, however, about its safety in pregnancy. This highlights the problems about drawing conclusions from uncontrolled data since both retrospective[12 13] and prospective[14 15] studies did not confirm any teratogenic effect. In the United States, the Food and Drugs Administration also concluded that there was no firm evidence linking this preparation with birth defects.[16] Nevertheless, the manufacturers withdrew the drug in 1983 because of the unsubstantiated claims about teratogenicity.[13]

21

Antihistamines

Antihistamines are generally recommended for treating nausea and vomiting in pregnancy.[17-19] Meclozine and cyclizine are widely used and appear to be safe. Concern about an association between the use of these drugs and congenital malformations, particularly cleft palate, has not been substantiated in prospective controlled studies.[20 21] There may, however, be a weak association between meclozine and congenital eye defects.[21] Promethazine may be associated with an increased incidence of congenital dislocation of the hips.[10 22]

Metoclopramide

Data on the effects of metoclopramide on early fetal development are lacking. It has been used in late pregnancy and in the management of hyperemesis gravidarum.[23] Since it increases lower oesophageal sphincter pressure and accelerates gastric emptying metoclopramide has been used in labour and before anaesthesia,[24] when it is considered safe and efficacious. Its routine use in early pregnancy cannot be recommended, however, because of the lack of controlled data.

Treatment of heartburn and dyspepsia

Heartburn due to gastro-oesophageal reflux is extremely common during pregnancy, particularly in the second and third trimesters. Lower oesophageal sphincter pressure is reduced throughout pregnancy and is lowest around the 36th week.[25]

Patients with symptoms of reflux should be reassured and advised to take small, frequent meals rich in carbohydrates and to avoid stooping or lying flat. If drug treatment is necessary teratogenicity is a less important issue because most cases start in late pregnancy. Non-absorbable antacids such as aluminium hydroxide or magnesium trisilicate may be used, although aluminium antacids given alone may cause constipation. Antacids are safe when taken in the second or third trimester, although they have been associated with an increased rate of congenital defects when taken in early pregnancy.[19] Metoclopramide, which raises lower oesophageal sphincter pressure, may be helpful in the management of reflux; its use in late pregnancy seems to be safe.[23][24]

Dyspepsia that is not related to oesophageal reflux is unusual in pregnancy. In particular, peptic ulcer rarely presents for the first time during pregnancy. In women with existing peptic ulcer symptoms tend to improve as the pregnancy progresses, but some may still require treatment. Simple measures include cessation of smoking, small regular meals, and antacids for relief of symptoms.

The H2-receptor antagonists cimetidine and ranitidine are safe and effective for managing peptic ulcer in non-obstetric practice. Routine use in pregnancy cannot, however, be recommended because of the lack of appropriate data on their safety. There is no justification for their use in the treatment of dyspepsia not related to ulceration since they are not even particularly effective.[26] H2-antagonists have been successfully used before general anaesthesia for caesarean section to reduce gastric acidity and prevent aspiration of acid into the lungs (Mendelson's syndrome). Both cimetidine and ranitidine are excreted into breast milk, but there are no data to suggest a harmful effect on the baby.

Sucralfate has not been widely used during pregnancy in the United Kingdom, but it is an effective treatment for peptic ulcer and has been recommended for use in pregnancy in the United States because it is not absorbed.[27] It may, however, cause mild constipation in some patients. Carbenoxolone causes salt and water retention and is therefore contraindicated in pregnancy. Compounds containing bismuth should also be avoided; the effects on fetal development of the absorption of small quantities of bismuth are unknown.

In summary, dyspepsia in pregnancy, whether related to peptic ulceration or not, is probably best managed with reassurance, advice on meals and smoking, and non-systemic antacids.

Treatment of constipation

Patients should be advised to take a diet high in cereal fibre and fresh fruit. Simple constipation is best treated by a bulking agent such as preparations containing bran, ispaghula, or methylcellulose. Stimulant laxatives may be uterotonic and are therefore contraindicated during pregnancy.

TREATMENT OF COMMON MINOR AILMENTS

Conclusions

It is a counsel of perfection that no drugs should be used in pregnancy, but some minor symptoms of common ailments often require treatment for the comfort of the mother. Paracetamol appears to be the safest minor analgesic; an antihistamine compound can probably be safely prescribed for a short period for treating nausea and vomiting; and heartburn and dyspepsia are best managed along simple lines, with an antacid in early pregnancy and possibly metoclopramide in the later stages.

1 Warkany J, Takacs E. Experimental productions of congenital malformation in rats by salicylate poisoning. *Am J Pathol* 1959;35:315–31.
Richards JD. Congenital malformations and environmental influences in pregnancy. *Br J Prev Soc Med* 1969;23:218–25.
3 Slone D, Siskind V, Heinonen OP, *et al*. Aspirin and congenital malformations. *Lancet* 1976;i:1373–5.
4 Turner G, Collins E. Foetal effects of regular salicylate ingestion in pregnancy. *Lancet* 1975;ii:338–9.
5 Shapiro S, Siskind V, Monson RR, *et al*. Perinatal mortality and birth-weight in relation to aspirin taken during pregnancy. *Lancet* 1976;i:1375–6.
6 Garrettson LK, Procknal JA, Levy G. Fetal acquisition and neonatal elimination of a large amount of salicylate. Study of a neonate whose mother regularly took therapeutic doses of aspirin during pregnancy. *Clin Pharmacol Ther* 1975;17:98–103.
7 Stuart MJ, Gross SJ, Elrad H, Graeber JE. Effects of acetylsalicylic-acid ingestion on maternal and neonatal hemostasis. *N Engl J Med* 1982;307:909–12.
8 Lubawy WC, Burris-Garrett RJ. Effects of aspirin and acetaminophen on fetal and placental growth in rats. *J Pharm Sci* 1977;66:111–3.
9 de Swiet M. *Medical disorders in obstetric practice*. Oxford: Blackwell Scientific, 1984.
10 Kullander S, Kallen B. A prospective study of drugs and pregnancy. II. Antiemetics. *Acta Obstet Gynecol Scand* 1976;55:105–11.
11 Klebanoff MA, Mills JL. Is vomiting during pregnancy teratogenic? *Br Med J* 1986;292:724–6.
12 Harron DWG, Griffiths K, Shanks RG. Debendox and congenital malformations in Northern Ireland. *Br Med J* 1980;281:1379–81.
13 Zierler S, Ruthman KJ. Congenital heart disease in relation to maternal use of benedictin and other drugs in early pregnancy. *N Engl J Med* 1985;313:347–52.
14 Milkovich LM, Van der Berg BJ. An evaluation of the teratogenicity of certain antinauseant drugs. *Am J Obstet Gynecol* 1976;125:244–8.
15 Smithells RW, Sheppard S. Teratogenicity testing in humans: a method of demonstrating safety of Benedictin. *Teratology* 1978;17:31.
16 Food and Safety Administration. *Federal Register* 1979;44:41068.
17 Lewis PJ, Chamberlain GVP. Treatment of everyday complaints in pregnancy. *Prescribers' Journal* 1982;22:77–84.
18 Fagan EA, Chadwick VS. Drug treatment of gastrointestinal disorders in pregnancy. In: Lewis PJ, ed. *Clinical pharmacology in obstetrics*. Bristol: Wright, 1983:114–37.
19 Nelson MM, Forfar JO. Associations between drugs administered during pregnancy and congenital abnormalities of the foetus. *Br Med J* 1971;i:523–7.
20 Smithells RW, Chinn ER. Meclozine and foetal malformation: a prospective study. *Br Med J* 1964;i:217–8.
21 Shapiro S, Kauffman DW, Rosenberg L, *et al*. Meclozine in pregnancy in relation to congenital malformations. *Br Med J* 1978;i:487.
22 Huff PS. Safety of drug therapy for nausea and vomiting of pregnancy. *J Fam Pract* 1980;11:969–70.

23 Singh MS, Lean TH. The use of metoclopramide in hyperemesis gravidarum. *Proceedings of the Obstetrics and Gynecology Society of Singapore* 1970;1:43.
24 Howard FA, Sharp DS. Effect of metoclopramide on gastric emptying in labour. *Br Med J* 1973;i:446–8.
25 Van Thiel DH, Gavaler JS, Joshi SN, Stremple J. Heartburn of pregnancy. *Gastroenterology* 1977;72:666–8.
26 Nyren O, Adami H-O, Bates S, Bergstrom R, Gustavsson S, Nyberg A. Absence of therapeutic benefit from antacids or cimetidine in non-ulcer dyspepsia. *N Engl J Med* 1986;324:339–43.
27 Lewis JH, Weingold AB. The use of gastrointestinal drugs during pregnancy and lactation. *Am J Gastroenterol* 1985;80:912–21.

Antibiotics

RICHARD WISE

Young women often develop infections, particularly of the urinary tract. Therefore pregnant women commonly require antimicrobial treatment. Bacteriuria occurs in about 5% of pregnancies, and if it is not treated between a quarter and a third of patients may develop pyelonephritis with consequent danger to their own health and an increased incidence of fetal loss.[1] Because pregnant women are often in an environment with young children they are at greater risk of developing the more trivial upper respiratory infections, which may require treatment. Occasionally, pregnant women need treatment for more serious infections. It is therefore necessary to know which antimicrobial agents can be used with negligible risk for the minor infections and to have some appreciation of the balance of risks for more serious cases.

In assessing the risk to the fetus several points should be considered. For many antimicrobial agents we now have more than 25 years' experience of freedom from congenital abnormality. Many studies have been performed in animals, but, although important, their results should be viewed with some reservation. For example, sulphonamides can cause gross fetal malformations when given in high doses to mice and rats,[2] but 50 years of use would surely have shown a teratogenic propensity in humans, which, to my knowledge, has not been recorded. One of the reasons why laboratory animals make poor models for studying fetal damage is the profound effect large doses of antimicrobial agents have on the animal's gastrointestinal flora and consequently on the animal's metabolism. On the other hand, certain drugs should definitely be avoided. For example, streptomycin causes neonatal ototoxicity after long term treatment of maternal tuberculosis.[3][4] It therefore follows, by implication rather than by hard information, that the other aminoglycosides, such as gentamicin, tobramycin, netilmicin, and amikacin, should be avoided for minor infections. In the treatment of serious maternal infection, however, their undoubted efficacy should be balanced against these theoretical risks.

Pregnant and non-pregnant women differ considerably in the way in which they handle antimicrobial agents, and this may influence treatment. Philipson showed that serum concentrations of ampicillin in women who were 9–36 weeks' pregnant were half the values found in the same women when they were not pregnant.[5] Low maternal concentrations have been described after ingestion of most antimicrobial agents, including aminoglycosides. The therapeutic implications of these low concentrations are difficult to assess. Failure of antibiotic treatment might incorrectly be blamed on the wrong choice of antibiotic and the drug might be replaced by a potentially more toxic agent. This could be particularly dangerous when treating a serious infection with an agent such as an aminoglycoside, when the natural caution of the doctor against giving what he might consider to be high doses will in fact cause more problems. In general, full adult doses should be used when treating infections in pregnant women. When serious infections are to be treated with an aminoglycoside, for example, assays should be performed to ensure that the patient is receiving sufficient drug and that neither she nor her fetus is being exposed to unacceptably high levels. Similarly, the length of treatment should be dictated by the disease and not be influenced unduly by the fact that the patient is pregnant. Inadequate treatment, which may be followed by further courses of antibiotics, is likely to put mother and fetus at greater risk than a full course of the correct antimicrobial agent. In the case of bacteriuria in pregnancy a 7–14 day course of treatment is usually prescribed, but some investigations suggest a single dose[6 7] or high dose short course.[8]

Antimicrobial agents

Table I lists various antimicrobial agents together with their possible toxic effects on the fetus in early or late pregnancy. I have attempted to give a safety rating: "probably safe" indicates that no significant risk to the fetus has been documented and hence such agents constitute a first choice if an antimicrobial agent has to be used; "caution" indicates that effects on the fetus have been

TABLE I—*Antimicrobial agents and their possible adverse effects*

Agent	Use	Adverse effects on the fetus		Comments
		First trimester	Second and third trimesters	
Penicillin (benzylpenicillin and phenoxymethylpenicillin)	Probably safe		Allergy; possibility of sensitising the fetus	All the commoner β lactams may be described as safe
Long acting penicillins	Probably safe		Allergy; possibility of sensitising the fetus	Little information available but no suggestion of increased toxicity
Ampicillin	Probably safe		Allergy; possibility of sensitising the fetus	Little information available. Reasonable to avoid prodrug formulation and use the parent ampicillin
Ampicillin prodrugs: Talampicillin, pivampicillin, bacampicillin				
Amoxycillin	Probably safe		Allergy; possibility of sensitising the fetus	
Amoxycillin and clavulanic acid (Augmentin)	Probably safe		Allergy; possibility of sensitising the fetus	Little information available. Best avoid until more experience reported
Antipseudomonal penicillins: Carbenicillin, mezlocillin, azlocillin, ticarcillin, piperacillin	Probably safe		Allergy; possibility of sensitising the fetus	Little information available. Reserve for treatment of serious infections caused by susceptible bacteria
Mecillinam	Probably safe		Allergy; possibility of sensitising the fetus	Little information available. Reserve for treatment of serious infections caused by susceptible bacteria
Antistaphylococcal penicillins: Flucloxacillin and cloxacillin	Probably safe		Allergy; possibility of sensitising the fetus	Little information available
Cephalosporins: Oral—cephalexin, cefaclor, cephradine	Probably safe		Allergy; possibility of sensitising the fetus	
Injectable	Probably safe		Allergy; possibility of sensitising the fetus	Little information available. These agents are probably safe and might well be reasonable choices in treatment of severe infection. Agents containing N-methyl tetrazole side should be avoided on theoretical grounds—that is, interference with vitamin K metabolism (latamoxef and cefamandole in the United Kingdom)

28

Drug	Safety in pregnancy	Fetal/neonatal risk	Comment
All agents	Probably safe in first trimester. Avoid within two days of delivery	Avoid (within two days of delivery), kernicterus	Risk is greater for more highly protein bound agents, such as sulphafurazole, rather than sulphamethoxazole
Trimethoprim	Probably safe		Theoretical teratogenic risk of folic acid antagonist. Risk of megaloblastic anaemia preventable by folinic acid
Co-trimoxazole (trimethoprim and sulphamethoxazole)	Probably safe (but see sulphonamide above)	Kernicterus	Considerable experience of safety in first trimester
Tetracyclines: All agents	Avoid	Discoloration and dysplasia of teeth and bones, cataracts	Possible hepatotoxicity in mother
Aminoglycosides: Streptomycin	Avoid	Ototoxicity	Little reason to be used. A better choice can be made in tuberculosis and serious sepsis
Gentamicin, tobramycin, netilmicin, amikacin	Caution	Theoretical risk of ototoxicity suggested	Effective in serious sepsis; regular assay required
Spectinomycin	Probably safe		Reserve for treatment of gonorrhoea when pencillin resistance or allergy is a problem
Fusidic acid	Probably safe		
Quinolones: Nalidixic acid	Caution		Wide experience suggests safety. Deposition in growing bones in certain animals. Interferes with bacterial DNA; theoretical risk to humans
Recently developed drugs: Ciprofloxacin, norfloxacin, enoxacin, ofloxacin, pefloxacin	Avoid		No experience in pregnancy—see nalidixic acid
Nitrofurantoin	Probably safe		Theoretical risk of haemolysis in glucose-6-phosphate dehydrogenase deficiency

TABLE I (CONTINUED)—*Antimicrobial agents and their possible adverse effects*

Agent	Use	Adverse effects on the fetus		Comments
		First trimetser	Second and third trimesters	
Vancomycin	Caution			Safety data not available in humans. Reserve for treatment of serious staphylococcal sepsis
Macrolides and lincosamides:				
Erythromycin base stearate	Probably safe			
Erythromycin estolate	Avoid			Maternal hepatotoxicity in late pregnancy
Lincomycin and clindamycin	Avoid			Maternal pseudomembranous colitis. Avoid unless no other suitable agent available
Metronidazole	Caution	Theoretical risk of teratogenesis		No evidence of teratogenicity in man. Benefit will probably outweigh risk in serious anaerobic sepsis
Chloramphenicol	Avoid		Grey baby syndrome	Little evidence of ill effect to fetus in early pregnancy. Remember possible maternal blood dyscrasias. Usually a safer choice can be made
Antituberculous agents:				
Rifampicin	Caution		Postnatal bleeding	Avoid in mothers with liver disease. High dosage teratogenicity in animals. Benefits probably outweigh risks. Vitamin K should be given to mother and neonate
Isoniazid	Probably safe			Observe mother for jaundice
Ethambutol	Probably safe			Now little used
Para-aminosalicylic acid	Probably safe			Little information available
Pyrazinamide	Caution			
Antifungal agents:				
Amphotericin	Caution			Limited information; safety not established
Flucytosine	Avoid	Teratogenic in animals		
Ketoconazole	Caution			Limited information; safety not established

Drug	Recommendation	Risk	Comments
Miconazole	Caution		Absorbed from vaginal topical use
Griseofulvin	Avoid	Teratogenic in animals	
Nystatin (topical)	Probably safe		
Antimalarial drugs:			
Chloroquine	Probably safe		Safety established in low dose, except for rare reports of hearing loss in children
Quinine	Avoid	Possible abortifacient	
Proguanil	Probably safe		
Pyrimethamine and dapsone (Maloprim)	Avoid		Teratogenicity reported in rats, but no convincing evidence in humans. Maloprim and Fansidar have been associated with fatalities
Pyrimethamine and sulpha-doxine (Fansidar)	Avoid		
Primaquine	Avoid		
Antiparasitic agents:			
Piperazine	Probably safe		
Mebendazole	Avoid	Possibly teratogenic	
Thiabendazole	Caution		
Praziquantrel	Caution		
Antiviral agents:			
Amantadine	Avoid	Embryotoxic in animals	Unless there is a life threatening infection in the mother it is probably best to avoid antiviral agents in pregnancy
Acyclovir	Caution	Theoretical risk	
Vidarabine	Avoid	Teratogenic in animals	

recorded with the agent (or a chemically related compound) or that its mode of action suggests a theoretical risk, but there may well be times when the balance of risks suggests that such compounds should be used. "Avoid" indicates that the agent carries a definite risk and its use might imply negligence (unless there was an overwhelming reason to the contrary). Such division of the compounds is obviously somewhat subjective.

Treatment of common conditions

Table II lists some of the common infections likely to be encountered in pregnancy. The first choice of treatment is usually an agent listed as probably safe in table I, although not necessarily so. A second choice agent might have to be used if (a) the patient is allergic to a first choice compound or (b) the bacteria responsible are resistant to the first choice agent. In this context it is particularly important to take cultures from pregnant patients before treatment so that a safe and efficacious change can be made to treatment if the patient does not respond or the causative organism proves resistant to initial treatment. The dose chosen should be that indicated for the condition in the *British National Formulary* and the clinician should eschew the temptation to use too low a dose. If the infection needs treating at all it needs full dosage.

Urinary tract infection

The most common reason for pregnant women to take antibiotics is for acute cystitis or covert bacteriuria. The choice of treatment is between ampicillin (or its close relative amoxycillin) and cephalexin (as the oral cephalosporin with which there is more experience). Cephalexin is probably more suitable because about one third of the common Gram negative bacteria which cause urinary tract infections are resistant to ampicillin. Although a combination of amoxycillin and clavulanic acid (Augmentin) has been used in pregnancy and it would overcome the problem of resistance, this combination might best be reserved for difficult cases until more evidence about its safety has accumulated. Women who are allergic to β lactams can be given a short course of trimethoprim with or without sulphamethoxazole in the first, and probably the second, trimester; in the third trimester nitrofurantoin would be an acceptable alternative.

Pharyngitis and tonsillitis

Most sore throats are caused by viruses and are therefore not susceptible to treatment. Patients with signs of systemic infection such as tachycardia, fever, and enlarged cervical lymph nodes should be given penicillin. If the infection is severe this should be given parenterally followed by phenoxymethylpenicillin. Patients allergic to penicillin should receive erythromycin base.

Bronchial and pulmonary infections

An acute bacterial bronchial infection after a viral bronchitis is not uncommon in a previously healthy young woman. The first choice of treatment is either ampicillin or amoxycillin. A specimen for culture should be taken, however, because 5-10% of *Haemophilus influenzae* are resistant to these two drugs. If the patient fails to respond this might be a reasonable indication for a course of treatment with a combination of amoxycillin and clavulanic acid.

The commonest cause of lobar pneumonia in a previously well young woman is *Streptococcus pneumoniae*, and this should be treated with benzylpenicillin, or erythromycin if the patient is allergic to benzylpenicillin. Legionnaires' disease is a common cause of community acquired pneumonia. There is still some doubt about the best treatment for this condition, but present knowledge suggests erythromycin. In seriously ill patients rifampicin may be added; however, this agent does not have a licence in the United Kingdom for legionella infections.

Surgical prophylaxis

Although elective operations are avoided in pregnancy, emergency operations may be necessary. The same guidelines for the choice of the correct prophylactic antibiotic should be followed—namely, that a short course of an appropriate agent should be given. If there is no evidence of established intra-abdominal sepsis (such as an appendix abscess) one to three doses of a parenteral cephalosporin such as cefuroxime plus metronidazole should be

TABLE II—*Common infectious conditions in pregnancy with recommended treatment*

Condition	First choice treatment	Second choice treatment	Comments
Asymptomatic bacteriuria or simple cystitis	Ampicillin, amoxycillin (if isolate sensitive), or cephalexin by mouth	Nitrofurantoin, sulphonamide, or trimethoprim (or co-trimoxazole)	In asymptomatic bacteriuria treatment should probably last 7-10 days Simple acute cystitis may respond to a single dose or short course
Acute pyelonephritis	Cefuroxime, ampicillin intravenously (if isolate sensitive)	Gentamicin intravenously	
Pharyngitis	Benzylpenicillin intravenously, procaine penicillin intramuscularly, or phenoxymethylpenicillin by mouth	Erythromycin base	Note: 70-80% of cases of pharyngitis are caused by viruses
Bronchitis	Ampicillin by mouth or amoxycillin	Erythromycin	
Lobar pneumonia	Benzylpenicillin	Erythromycin	If not pneumococcal change in treatment may be required
Legionnaires' disease	Erythromycin plus rifampicin		
Endocarditis prophylaxis	Amoxycillin by mouth	Erythromycin	Follow recommendations of working party[8]
Endocarditis treatment: Streptococcal Staphylococcal	Benzylpenicillin + gentamicin Flucloxacillin + fusidic acid	Vancomycin	

TABLE II (CONTINUED)—*Common infectious conditions in pregnancy with recommended treatment*

Gonorrhoea	Benzylpenicillin intramuscularly	Cefuroxime or spectinomycin	Spectinomycin if patient is β-lactam allergic
Infection caused by *Chlamydia trachomatis*	Erythromycin by mouth		Erythromycin should be given for 7-10 days
Prophylaxis for abdominal operations: Gastric or biliary Appendicectomy or colonic	1 dose cefazolin 1-3 doses amoxycillin and clavulanic acid (Augmentin)	1 dose co-trimoxazole 1-3 doses gentamicin plus metronidazole	
Tuberculosis	Rifampicin + isoniazid + ethambutol		Rifampicin and isoniazid should be given for 9 months and ethambutol for 3 months. Pyridoxine supplements should be given with isoniazide
Malaria prophylaxis	Chloroquine		See text
Serious undiagnosed sepsis	Gentamicin intravenously + antipseudomonal penicillin intravenously, possibly plus metronidazole	Broad spectrum cephalosporin intravenously (such as cefuroxime or ceftazidime)	On establishing causative pathogen it may be possible to omit gentamicin if (*a*) organisms susceptible to antipseudomonal penicillin and (*b*) patient has made a satisfactory response

given (or possibly cefoxitin or amoxycillin and clavulanic acid alone). If there is abscess formation then three to four days' treatment is required.

For patients who need antibiotic prophylaxis because of a pre-existing heart disorder the guidelines of the British Society for Antimicrobial Chemotherapy working party should be followed.

Septicaemia

Happily, it is rare to have to treat a pregnant patient with a microbiologically undiagnosed possible septicaemia. In such instances the risks to the patient outweigh the risks to the fetus and broad spectrum antimicrobial agents in full dosage should be prescribed. Parenteral cefuroxime would be a good first choice, possibly with the addition of metronidazole if there is evidence of intra-abdominal sepsis. Once a pathogen and its antimicrobial susceptibilities have been determined treatment can be directed at that organism.

Tuberculosis

Because of the chronic nature of tuberculosis it is not uncommon to encounter this infection in pregnancy. Young women who are not pregnant should be warned of the increased risk of failure of the contraceptive pill if, as is likely, rifampicin is prescribed.

Opinions differ on the treatment of infections with *Mycobacteria tuberculosis* in pregnant women. This difference is mainly concerned with the risks associated with rifampicin, which readily crosses the placenta; teratogenicity has been suggested but not confirmed. Treatment should not be appreciably different from that in non-pregnant patients and should be of full duration. Streptomycin is rarely used in tuberculosis and should certainly be avoided in pregnant women. Treatment by a physician who specialises in respiratory medicine is advisable.

Malaria prophylaxis and treatment

Malaria is an important cause of abortion, premature labour, and perinatal death, as well as affecting the mother. Hence both prophylaxis and treatment are required during pregnancy. Prophylaxis should be started one week before visiting a malarial area and continued for one month after leaving. For travel to north Africa and the Middle East, where chloroquine resistance has not been reported, chloroquine 300 mg weekly is advised. Travel to a country where chloroquine resistant *P falciparum* is found presents a problem. Pyrimethamine and sulfadoxine (Fansidar) and pyrimethamine and dapsone (Maloprim) are now considered to carry sufficient risk of Stevens-Johnson syndrome and neutropenia respectively to almost outweigh their benefits, not only in pregnant women but in any individual. Pregnant women should be advised not to visit an area where chloroquine resistant *P falciparum* is found (such as east and central Africa, South East Asia, and South America). For women who intend to visit a major urban centre only (where the risk is smaller) chloroquine 300 mg a week plus proguanil 200 mg a day should be prescribed.

In the treatment of benign malaria (caused by *P vivax*, *P ovale*, and *P malaraie*) chloroquine should be used; radical cure with primaquine should not be undertaken until after pregnancy to avoid the possibility of haemolysis due to glucose-6-phosphate dehydrogenase deficiency. *P falciparum* malaria should again be treated with chloroquine except when the patient comes from an area where chloroquine resistance is known. In such cases quinine should be used. Quinine will reduce the numbers of parasites in the blood and after a three day course a single dose of three tablets of Fansidar is warranted. Then, if asexual parasites are still present in a blood smear a seven day course of erythromycin should be given.

Other parasitic infections

Toxoplasmosis—Fetal infection in the first trimester is relatively uncommon, but in most of the cases that do occur the disease is severe. In the last trimester, however, infection of the fetus by an infected mother is more usual, but most babies will have no overt disease at birth. The treatment suggested is as follows: pyrimethamine 50 mg twice weekly, plus folic acid 5 mg daily, plus sulphadiazine 50 mg/kg twice daily. Patients should have treatment for two weeks followed by four weeks without treatment; this should be repeated throughout pregnancy. Anyone considering treating a pregnant patient with possible toxoplasmosis should liaise with an expert in this disease.

Amoebiasis—Metronidazole 800 mg three times daily should be given for five days followed by diloxanide furonate 500 mg three times daily for five days (to eliminate trophozoites from the gut lumen).

Giardiasis—Metronidazole 400 mg three times daily should be given for seven days. Relapses are not uncommon.

Helminthiasis—Most infections with ascaris and trichuris are asymptomatic and are best left alone in pregnancy. Occasionally, a 4 g dose of piperazine may be required. Heavy hookworm infections should be treated with 5 g of bephenium or 10 mg/kg of prantel pamoate if anaemia is severe.

Venereal diseases

As penicillin forms the basis of the treatment of both gonorrhoea and syphilis there is no need for any change in treatment in pregnancy, and both conditions should be treated vigorously and followed up (in both mother and infant). A problem can arise in the treatment of syphilis in pregnant women who are allergic to penicillin. It is doubtful if erythromycin is satisfactory in eradicating spirochaetes from the fetus. In such cases it might be reasonable to use tetracycline because the effect of congenital syphilis on the teeth (not to mention other sites) would be more severe than the effect of tetracycline. Chlamydial infections causing non-specific urethritis during pregnancy should be treated with erythromycin.

Pelvic inflammatory disease

Pelvic inflammatory disease is not uncommon in pregnancy, and treatment is difficult. Patients should be given erythromycin together with metronidazole (except in the first trimester).

Antibiotics and lactation

Both mother and general practitioner are often anxious that antimicrobial agents being used to treat the mother are being transferred to the infant. Although most antibiotics are found in breast milk in low concentrations, they are unlikely to affect the child. This is because appreciable amounts of the agent will not be absorbed from the infant's gastrointestinal tract—for example, the aminoglycosides and injectable cephalosporins—or, if the agents are absorbed, the concentrations reached in the infant are extremely low—for example, ampicillins. Concern has been expressed, however, over a few agents.

Chloramphenicol—Although grey baby syndrome is most unlikely (as concentrations are too low), the possibility of infant marrow toxicity necessitates either avoiding this agent or stopping breast feeding.

Tetracyclines—Tetracyclines should be avoided because of the theoretical, rather than real, risk of teeth discoloration. Chelation of the tetracycline by the calcium ions in milk probably overcomes this problem.

Sulphonamides (including co-trimoxazole)—Although the risk of kernicterus is low, it should be borne in mind especially if a highly protein bound sulphonamide—for example, sulphadimethoxine— is being used. In glucose-6-phosphate dehydrogenase deficiency there is the risk of haemolytic anaemia.

Isoniazid—There is a theoretical risk of convulsions with isoniazid. Both mother and baby should be given pyridoxine.

Metronidazole—Mothers who start taking metronidazole after they have started breast feeding may find that it has an adverse effect on the taste of the milk.

Conclusion

A wide range of antimicrobial agents is now available and harmful effects on the fetus have been proved in relatively few. Infection in pregnant women usually requires treatment and the choice of agent should not be a major problem.

1 Condie AP, Brumfitt W, Reeves DS, Williams JD. The effects of bacteriuria in pregnancy on foetal health. In: Brumfitt W, Asscher AW, eds. *Urinary tract infection*. London: Oxford University Press, 1973.
2 Kato T, Kitagawa S. Production of congenital abnormalities in fetuses of rats and mice with various sulphonamides. *Congenital Abnormalities* 1973;13:7–15.
3 Assael BM, Parini R, Rusconi F. Ototoxicity of aminoglycoside antibiotics in infants and children. *Pediatr Infect Dis* 1982;1:357–67.
4 Conway N, Birt BD. Streptomycin in pregnancy: effect on the foetal ear. *Br Med J* 1965;ii:260–3.

5 Philipson A. Pharmacokinetics of antibiotics in pregnancy and labour. *Clin Pharmacokinet* 1979;4:297–309.

6 Harris RE, Gilstrap LC, Pretty A. Single dose antimicrobial therapy for asymptomatic bacteriuria during pregnancy. *Obstet Gynecol* 1982;59:546.

7 Bailey RR, Bishop V, Reddie BA. Comparison of single dose with a 5 day course of co-trimoxazole for asymptomatic (covert) bacteriuria in pregnancy. *Aust N Z J Obstet Gynaecol* 983;23:41.

8 Anderstan KJ, Abbas AMA, Davey A, Ancill RJ. High dose, short course amoxycillin in the treatment of bacteriuria in pregnancy. *Br J Clin Prac* 1983;37:212–4.

9 Working Party of the British Society for Antimicrobial Chemotherapy. The antibiotic prophylaxis of endocarditis. *Lancet* 1982;ii:1323–6.

Treatment of asthma

K FAN CHUNG, PETER J BARNES

About 1% of pregnant women suffer from active asthma.[1-3] Current evidence suggests that uncontrolled asthma may lead to maternal hypoxaemia with potentially grave consequences for the fetus. Asthma in pregnancy should therefore be treated promptly and appropriately to reduce perinatal mortality and morbidity. As in non-obstetric practice, management of pregnant women with asthma aims at preventing recurrent attacks of wheezing, status asthmaticus, and respiratory failure. Drugs that are teratogenic or detrimental to the fetus should obviously be avoided.

Asthma and pregnancy

Pulmonary function during pregnancy

The enlarging fetus and the increased concentrations of circulating hormones, such as progesterone and cortisol, contribute to several changes in pulmonary function in pregnancy.[4-7] Reductions in residual volume and functional residual capacity occur before appreciable enlargement of the uterus. Spirometric tests of airway function such as forced expiratory volume in one second remain unchanged. Throughout pregnancy there is a progressive rise in minute ventilation, mostly due to an increased tidal volume, and arterial blood gas measurements reflect a compensated respiratory alkalosis. The partial pressure of arterial oxygen remains normal or is slightly increased. These changes have no effect on the course of asthma or on the fetus.

Fetal oxygenation

Maternal hypoxaemia and respiratory alkalosis, which may

result during an acute attack of asthma, are detrimental to the fetus, particularly during the first trimester. The fetus exists in relative hypoxaemia with an umbilical venous pressure of oxygen of 4·3 kPa (32 mm Hg).[8] This is compensated for by the fact that fetal haemoglobin binds more avidly to oxygen and releases it more efficiently in tissues. Fetal partial pressure of oxygen is adequately maintained provided inspired maternal oxygen is at least 7%, but the fetus has a reserve of oxygen lasting only two minutes. Hypocapnia, to values of 2·3 kPa (17 mm Hg) or less, may substantially depress fetal oxygen values and may be associated with clinically depressed infants at birth.[9] Hypocapnia causes constriction of the uterine arteries with subsequent reduction in placental blood flow and increases the affinity of maternal haemoglobin for oxygen.[8]

Effect of pregnancy on asthma

A review of several retrospective and uncontrolled studies showed that in half of 1054 pregnancies patients reported no change in their asthma, 29% improved, and 21% became worse.[10] The severity of asthma before pregnancy seems to determine the course during pregnancy. Thus patients with severe asthma before pregnancy tend to become worse during pregnancy and those with mild asthma usually show little change[11]; subsequent pregnancies show a similar pattern.

Effect of asthma on pregnancy and the fetus

One study showed that mothers with asthma had a higher incidence of maternal complications, such as pre-eclampsia, during pregnancy than a control group of pregnant women.[12] There is also a higher incidence of perinatal mortality in infants of asthmatic mothers, and a slight increase in the incidence of premature births.[2 12] In a study of 55 women with asthma severe enough to require treatment with oral corticosteroids during their pregnancies the incidence of maternal and fetal morbidity and mortality was not increased when compared with that of a control group.[13] This study suggested that adequate control of asthma may prevent the effects of asthma on pregnancy and on the fetus.

Drug treatment of asthma during pregnancy

The main classes of antiasthmatic drugs are: (*a*) bronchodilators, such as β adrenergic agonists and theophyllines, and (*b*) prophylactic or anti-inflammatory agents such as corticosteroids (oral or inhaled) and sodium cromoglycate. Their use in pregnant women with asthma has been reviewed elsewhere.[10 14 15]

β Adrenoceptor agonists

β_2 Adrenoceptor agonists are extremely effective bronchodilator agents in asthma. They should be given as an aerosol and are the drugs of choice for treating episodic wheezing and acute asthmatic attacks during pregnancy. There are minimal maternal side effects such as tachycardia, nervousness, and muscle tremor.

Teratogenesis has not been reported with the β_2 adrenergic agonists such as salbutamol and terbutaline.[14 16] Both drugs probably cross the placenta but this has not been confirmed. Terbutaline is secreted in breast milk, but it was not detected in the breast fed baby of a mother given an oral dose of terbutaline.[17]

Adrenaline and isoprenaline are best avoided during pregnancy. Adrenaline crosses the placenta and, in large doses, may cause fetal tachycardia and vasoconstriction of the uteroplacental circulation. A slightly increased incidence of congenital malformation has been reported after use of adrenaline during pregnancy.[18] For similar reasons, ephedrine, which is only a mild bronchodilator, should not be used. Isoprenaline also crosses the human placenta and induces cardiac and aortic arch anomalies in chick embryo. These β adrenergic drugs can be easily replaced by the more selective β_2 adrenergic agonists.

Theophyllines

Theophylline preparations are less effective as bronchodilators than β_2 agonists but may have additive effects after they have been given in maximally effective doses. Theophylline may be added to maintenance treatment if adequate control of asthma is not achieved with an inhaled β_2 agonist and inhaled corticosteroid. Another common indication for theophylline is the control of nocturnal asthma and early morning wheeze.

Although theophylline has been reported to induce chromosome breaks in human lymphocytes in culture, congenital anomalies did not occur in 117 women taking the drug during the first trimester.[18] Theophylline crosses the placenta and attains similar concentrations in maternal and fetal circulations.[19] It also appears in the milk of mothers taking the drug with a milk to plasma ratio of about 0·7; the maximum concentration in milk occurs two hours after the peak serum concentration.[20] A breast fed baby has been estimated to receive less than 10% of the mother's dose. Tachycardia and transient jitteriness have been reported in three newborn infants whose mothers had blood concentrations of theophylline within the therapeutic range. Excessive irritability in breast fed infants of mothers receiving theophylline may be a sign of theophylline toxicity in the infant. Breast feeding before taking the scheduled dose of theophylline reduces neonatal exposure to the drug. No long term adverse effects have been reported in infants of mothers receiving theophylline throughout pregnancy.

There is limited information on the effects of pregnancy on theophylline pharmacokinetics. Blood concentrations of theophylline should be monitored to avoid underdosing or overdosing.

Corticosteroids

Corticosteroids are powerful, effective agents for the treatment of acute, severe attacks of asthma and of chronic asthma. Steroid aerosols give treatment equivalent to a substantial dose of oral steroids but avoid systemic side effects.

The safety of inhaled beclomethasone dipropionate has been evaluated in 45 pregnancies in 40 women with severe asthma taking a mean daily dose of 336 mg.[21] Beclomethasone aerosol was used regularly in 38 pregnancies from the time of conception. The risk of congenital malformations, spontaneous abortions, stillbirths, and neonatal deaths was within the normal range. In another study of 20 patients who become pregnant while taking an unstated dose of beclomethasone no congenital malformations or abortions were recorded.[22]

An increased incidence of cleft palate in the offspring of rabbits given cortisone acetate during pregnancy has been reported, but no increase in abnormalities was found in 145 infants exposed to corticosteroids during the first trimester of pregnancy.[18] Early reports linked prednisolone to an increased incidence of stillbirths and unexpected fetal distress due to placental insufficiency.[23] These findings have not been confirmed in more recent studies, however, which found no increased risk of spontaneous abortion, congenital malformations, stillbirths, neonatal deaths, pre-eclampsia, or bleeding in 70 pregnancies in 55 patients with asthma receiving a mean daily dose of prednisolone 8·2 mg.[13 24] There was a slight increase in the incidence of premature birth, but this effect could have resulted from other factors.

Cortisol and corticosteroids cross the placenta rapidly, and most of the cortisol is converted rapidly into inactive cortisone by fetal enzymes.[25] Dexamethasone crosses the placenta in high concentrations, achieving similar values in the fetus.[26] On the other hand, prednisolone is transferred slowly and the concentration of active compound in fetal blood is 10% of that in the mother.[27] Prednisolone equilibrates rapidly in the infant but is converted to the active prednisolone only slowly and is therefore functionally inactive in the fetus. It appears reasonable to prescribe either prednisone or prednisolone if steroids are to be used to treat asthmatic patients during pregnancy. Prednisone and prednisolone are secreted in breast milk in small amounts,[28 29] but a dose of less than 30 mg/day is unlikely to cause any problems in breast fed infants.

The incidence of hypoadrenalism in children of mothers taking corticosteroids is low, probably because of the widespread use of prednisolone or prednisone. Neonates whose mothers have taken prednisone throughout pregnancy have normal cortisol production.

Sodium cromoglycate

Sodium cromoglycate is a useful prophylactic agent in some young patients with atopic asthma. Large intravenous doses of sodium cromoglycate in rats and rabbits do not have any teratogenic effects, and results of one large study suggest that it is safe in pregnant women with asthma using the recommended inhaled dosage throughout pregnancy.[30] There are no data on the transfer of sodium cromoglycate across the placenta. Because it is poorly absorbed after inhalation[31] the amounts available for transfer across the placenta are insignificant.

Management of asthma in pregnant and nursing mothers

In common with several other medical complications of pregnancy the management of asthma should ideally begin before conception. Treatment should be optimised: if possible the number of drugs taken should be reduced and undesirable agents (such as antihistamines) discontinued. As with non-pregnant patients, the aim of treatment is to control and prevent acute episodes of asthma.

Measures such as avoiding allergens or known triggering factors and treatment of associated reflux oesophagitis and rhinitis or sinusitis may lead to an improvement in control. Treatment with β_2 agonist drugs in aerosol form is preferable to oral treatment, with a reduction in systemic side effects. Theophyllines should be added only when both inhaled β_2 agonists and corticosteroids fail to control asthma. Sodium cromoglycate may be useful in allergic asthmatics who have previously responded to it.

The treatment of acute severe episodes of asthma in pregnant patients is similar to that in non-pregnant patients. β_2 Agonists given by inhalation from a nebuliser and oral corticosteroids, preferably prednisolone or intravenous methylprednisolone, remain the drugs of choice. Arterial blood gases should be checked to avoid levels of hypocapnia and hypoxaemia which are detrimental to the fetus, and supplementary oxygen should be given. Intravenous theophylline may be added to the treatment of acute asthma when there is little or slow response to the combination of β_2 agonists and corticosteroid; serum theophylline concentrations should be monitored closely.

Maintenance treatment with oral or inhaled corticosteroids is indicated if repeated short courses of oral steroids are continually followed by relapse and if β_2 agonists fail to control symptoms. It is desirable to use single daily doses of prednisone and to change to inhaled corticosteroids such as beclomethasone dipropionate as soon as symptoms are controlled. Inhaled corticosteroids can usually be substituted in patients requiring low doses of maintenance oral corticosteroids. At the time of delivery patients previously treated with oral corticosteroids should be given hydrocortisone 100 mg every eight hours, starting at presentation and continuing for 24 hours after delivery.

There is no reason why an asthmatic mother who takes anti-asthmatic drugs should not breast feed her infant. In general a regimen of inhaled β_2 agonist, theophylline in the therapeutic range, and oral or inhaled corticosteroids should be safe and effective for the mother and baby.

1 Schaefer G, Silverman F. Pregnancy complicated by asthma. *Am J Obstet Gynecol* 1961;**82**:182–91.

2 Gordon M, Niswander KR, Berendes H, Kantor AG. Fetal morbidity following potentially anoxigenic obstetric conditions: VII. Bronchial asthma. *Am J Obst Gynecol* 1970;**106**:421–9.

3 de Swiet M. Diseases of the respiratory system. *Clin Obstet Gynaecol* 1977;**4**:287–96.

4 Gazioglu K, Kaltreider NL, Rosen M, Yu PN. Pulmonary function during pregnancy in normal women and in patients with cardiopulmonary disease. *Thorax* 1970;**25**:445–50.

5 Knuttgen HG, Emerson K. Physiological response to pregnancy at rest and at exercise. *J Appl Physiol* 1974;**36**:549–53.

6 Lim VS, Katz AI, Lindheimer MD. Acid-base regulation in pregnancy. *Am J Physiol* 1976;**231**:1764–70.

7 Milne JA. The respiratory response to pregnancy. *Postgrad Med J* 1979;**55**:318–24.

8 Wulf KH, Kunzel W, Lehmann V. Clinical aspects of placental gas exchange. In: Lango LD, Bartels H, eds. *Respiratory gas exchange and blood flow in the placenta*. Bethesda, Maryland: National Institute of Health, Public Health Service, US Department of Health, Education, and Welfare, 1972:505–21.

9 Moya F, Marishima HO, Shnider SM, James LS. Influence of maternal hyperventilation on the newborn infant. *Am J Obstet Gynecol* 1965;**91**:76–84.

10 Turner ES, Greenberger PA, Patterson R. Management of the pregnant asthmatic patient. *Ann Intern Med* 1980;**6**:905–18.

11 Gluck JC, Gluck PA. The effects of pregnancy on asthma: a prospective study. *Ann Allergy* 1976;**37**:164–8.

12 Bahna SL, Bjerkdal T. The cause and outcome of pregnancy in women with bronchial asthma. *Allergy* 1972;**27**:397–406.

13 Schatz M, Patterson R, Zeitz S, O'Rourke J, Melan H. Corticosteroid therapy for the pregnant asthmatic patient. *JAMA* 1975;**233**:804–7.

14 Romero R, Berkowitz R. The use of anti-asthmatic drugs in pregnancy. In: Niebyl JR, ed. *Drug use in pregnancy*. Philadelphia: Lea and Febiger, 1982:41–59.

15 Greenberger PA, Patterson R. Management of asthma during pregnancy. *N Engl J Med* 1985;**312**:897–902.

16 Mintz S. Pregnancy and asthma. In: Weiss EB, Segal MS, Stein M. eds. *Bronchial asthma, mechanisms and therapeutics*. 2nd ed. Boston: Little, Brown, 1985:878–91.

17 Lonnerholm G, Lindstrom B. Terbutaline excretion into breast milk. *Br J Clin Pharmacol* 1983;**13**:729–30.

18 Heinonen OP, Slone D, Shapiro S. *Birth defects and drugs in pregnancy*. Littleton: Publishing Sciences Group, 1977.

19 Labovitz E, Spector S. Placental theophylline transfer in pregnant asthmatics. *JAMA* 1982;**247**:768–8.

20 Yurchek AM, Jusko WJ. Theophylline secretion into breast milk. *Pediatrics* 1976;**57**:518.

21 Greenberger PA, Patterson R. Beclomethasone dipropionate for severe asthma during pregnancy. *Ann Intern Med* 1983;**98**:478–80.

22 Morrow-Brown H, Storey G. Beclomethasone dipropionate aerosol in long-term treatment of perennial and seasonal asthma in children and adults: a report of five and half years experience in 600 asthmatic patients. *Br J Clin Pharmacol* 1977;**4**:529S–67S.

23 Warrell DW, Taylor R. Outcome for the fetus of mothers receiving prednisolone during pregnancy. *Lancet* 1968;i:117–8.

24 Snyder RD, Snyder D. Corticosteroid for asthma during pregnancy. *Ann Allergy* 1978;**41**:340.

25 Murphy BE, Clark SJ, Donald IR, Pinsky M, Vedady D. Conversion of maternal cortisol to cortisone during placental transfer to the human foetus. *Am J Obstet Gynecol* 1974;**118**:538–41.

26 Osathanonsh A, Tulchinsky D, Kamali H, Fencl MD, Taeusch HW. Dexamethasone levels in treated pregnant women and newborn infants. *J Pediatr* 1977;**90**:617–20.

27 Beitins IZ, Bayard F, Ances IG, Kowaski A, Migem CJ. The transplacental passage of prednisone and prednisolone in pregnancy near term. *J Pediatr* 1972;**81**:936–45.

28 McKenzie SA, Sellers JA, Agnew JE. Secretion of prednisolone into breast milk. *Arch Dis Child* 1975;**50**:894–6.

29 Katz FH, Duncan BR. Entry of prednisone into human breast milk. *N Engl J Med* 1975;**292**:1154.

30 Wilson J. Utilisation du cromoglycate de sodium au cours de la grossesse. *Acta Therapeutica* 1982;**8**(suppl):45–51.

31 Walker SR, Richards AJ, Paterson JW. The absorption, excretion and metabolism of disodium (14ᶜ) cromoglycate in man. *Biochem J* 1971;**125**:27.

Psychotropic drugs

J B LOUDON

At some time during their pregnancy at least 10% of a random sample of women attending antenatal classes will experience appreciable psychological distress, mainly anxiety.[1] Of those who have suffered previous psychological illness or undergone termination of pregnancy the figure may be as high as 16%.[2] Few women are referred to a psychiatrist during pregnancy. During the puerperium 0·2% of mothers develop a psychotic illness, at least 10% develop a depressive illness, and a further 16% suffer a self limiting depressive reaction, qualitatively different from the "birth time blues," which lasts up to a month.[3] Often these depressive illnesses and reactions are not reported to the patient's general practitioner, but they are corrosive to personal well being and to marital happiness and merit both attention and appropriate treatment.

The distress of pregnancy may be related to adverse events or social circumstances, being more common in unmarried women, and it is probably less amenable to drug treatment. For the disorders of the puerperium, which seem to be caused by a biological disturbance but which occur more often in primigravidas, in the unmarried, in those who have undergone section, and after a perinatal death, drug treatment is likely to be indicated.[3a] This chapter discusses psychotropic drugs, but it should be remembered that other forms of treatment are important and include support from staff or self help groups, psychological treatments such as relaxation exercises or cognitive therapy, and mobilisation of community resources.

Psychotropic drugs used in pregnancy and during the puerperium will be dealt with in four groups: the hypnotic and anxiolytic drugs, neuroleptic drugs, antidepressants, and lithium carbonate.

49

Safety of psychotropic drugs used in pregnancy and during the puerperium

Hypnotic and anxiolytic drugs: benzodiazepines

Only benzodiazepine drugs should be used; barbiturates and the older anxiolytic drugs such as meprobamate are obsolete. Reports from Scandinavia in the early 1970s suggested greater use of benzodiazepines by the mothers of children born with defects of the palate, although other studies of the time failed to confirm the finding. Recently, a careful study which compared 611 infants with such deformities and 2498 controls found no evidence of an excess of diazepam use by their mothers.[4] Some reassurance can therefore be given to an anxious woman who has been taking diazepam in early pregnancy. Abrupt withdrawal of diazepam under these circumstances is not justified.

There is no evidence to suggest that benzodiazepines have a harmful effect on the fetus later in pregnancy, but the need for these drugs has to be clear to justify their use, especially on a regular basis. Diazepam appears in fetal blood within a few minutes of an intravenous or intramuscular injection, but the fetus seems to have a limited capacity to metabolise the drug.[5] Pharmacologically, the fetus acts as a "deep compartment," wherein diazepam is slow to accumulate but also, with its active metabolites, is eliminated slowly. This means that regular ingestion of diazepam by the mother will result in accumulation in the fetus. These factors appear to explain the finding that during labour a single bolus of less than 30 mg of diazepam has no adverse effect on the infant as measured by the Apgar score. A larger single dose or sustained prenatal benzodiazepine ingestion can lead to the "floppy infant syndrome," which is characterised by hypotonia, respiratory embarrassment, difficulty in suckling, and hypothermia. There is also good evidence for a withdrawal syndrome in infants whose mothers have taken benzodiazepines regularly during pregnancy.[6]

Diazepam is present in maternal blood un-ionised and is lipophilic; it is therefore readily transferred to breast milk. The newborn infant continues to have an impaired ability to metabolise the drug completely, and diazepam has been found in an infant six days after a single dose was given to the mother. Regular use by the mother leads to accumulation in the child. There is little justification for use by nursing mothers of diazepam or any other long acting, older, drugs such as chlordiazepoxide or nitrazepam. Lorazepam has been associated with neonatal hypotonicity but may not enter breast milk in troublesome amounts. Neonates seem to be able to metabolise oxazepam satisfactorily after the second or third day,[7] which might justify preference for this drug if a benzodiazepine has to be used by the nursing mother.

Neuroleptic drugs: phenothiazines and thioxanthines

Pregnant women are unlikely to start taking drugs in this group unless as an obsolete and inadvisable treatment for anxiety. A number of women who have suffered from episodes of a functional psychosis may, however, be on long term neuroleptic treatment as prophylaxis and may neglect contraceptive measures as a result of the illness or its after effects. A study of schizophrenic mothers showed that neonatal mortality is twice that of normal controls,[8] which makes assessment of the dangers of neuroleptic drugs more difficult. Several studies have failed to show a teratogenic effect of neuroleptic drugs, especially trifluoperazine, taken in early pregnancy,[9] and no lasting behavioural or developmental effects on the child have been found as a result of exposure to neuroleptic drugs in later pregnancy. Prochlorperazine, which is used more often as an antiemetic, has been shown to be teratogenic when the fetus is exposed between the sixth and 10th weeks of gestation.[10]

Neuroleptic drugs enter breast milk in clinically unimportant amounts. There are a few reports of a pseudoparkinsonian reaction in neonates born to mothers taking oral or depot neuroleptic drugs.[11]

Tricyclic antidepressants

There is a close structural relation between many neuroleptic drugs and the tricyclic antidepressants and much overlap in their pharmacological effects. Not surprisingly, therefore, the information about their use during pregnancy and lactation is similar.[12] The newer non-tricyclic antidepressants are a different matter in that their safety has not yet been proved. Given that two such drugs (zimelidine and nomifensine) have been withdrawn in the

51

past four years because of unexpected toxicity once they came into widespread use, these newer drugs are best avoided in pregnancy.

As happens in adults when tricyclic drugs are suddenly withdrawn, a withdrawal reaction has been reported in some neonates born to mothers who received tricyclic antidepressants in the last month of pregnancy.[13] The effects include irritability, apparent abdominal cramps, restlessness, insomnia, and fever.

Both neuroleptic drugs and tricyclic antidepressants enter breast milk in detectable quantities, but ingestion of small amounts of these drugs does not appear to affect the neonate. Indeed, follow up studies over long periods of the children of mothers taking chlorpromazine failed to show any adverse effect on development.[14] There is little published information on the transfer of monoamine oxidase inhibitors to breast milk; tranylcypromine appears to be safe for nursing mothers.[15]

Lithium carbonate

In some parts of the United Kingdom nearly one person in 1000 takes lithium as prophylaxis for recurrent affective illness; a substantial number of these are women of childbearing age. Many studies have confirmed the teratogenic effect of lithium taken in the first months of pregnancy. The cardiovascular system is usually affected, in particular the tricuspid valve (see previous chapter on identifying abnormalities). A recent study has confirmed previous figures of a 7% risk and given some valuable comparisons.[16] In a group of pregnant women suffering from manic depression the risk of fetal cardiac abnormalities was increased fivefold in those taking lithium compared with those taking other drugs. Nine of 59 children born to mothers taking lithium were malformed or died soon after birth compared with one of 38 taking drugs other than lithium.

Lithium clearance doubles during pregnancy, which may necessitate an increase in the total daily intake of lithium to maintain the same serum concentration. At the time of delivery the clearance abruptly falls back to normal, and this may be sufficiently fast to precipitate toxic concentrations of lithium in the mother. There is no evidence of a withdrawal reaction or behavioural abnormality in neonates exposed to lithium in utero.

Lithium enters breast milk freely, and serum concentrations in neonates may be close to values that are therapeutic in adults.[17] [18] Toxicity may therefore supervene if there is negative sodium or water balance in the infant.

Guidelines for drug use during pregnancy and in the puerperium

Patients already receiving treatment

The aim of minimising exposure of the fetus and the neonate to psychotropic drugs is helped enormously by patients who are educated and enlightened about treatment. Lines of management differ for those known to have suffered a psychological disorder before the particular pregnancy and those whose illness has arisen for the first time during pregnancy or in the puerperium.

Patients already receiving long term psychotropic treatment for psychosis should take contraceptive measures or, if no further children are wanted, should be offered sterilisation as the puerperium is a time of high risk of recurrence of a previous psychosis, with all that that implies for the progression of secondary and tertiary handicap. This issue should be discussed with both the patient and her partner, not once but several times, in language which is clear and non-technical to allow a satisfactory decision to be made. If such a patient is determined to conceive it will be a fine clinical decision whether to risk relapse by withdrawing psychotropic drugs or risk the slight possibility of fetal damage. The fetus may be harmed more by the effects of maternal relapse.

Patients receiving long term lithium prophylaxis are a particular problem if the question of another pregnancy is raised. A sudden desire for pregnancy may be a manifestation of a hypomanic mood swing, which is partially controlled with lithium carbonate. Immediate withdrawal of lithium may result in a full blown illness. The issue must be discussed with the couple over several sessions, which will enable the would be mother's mental state to be more fully assessed. If lithium is to be withdrawn it should be done gradually over six or eight weeks, and attempts at conception should be delayed to ensure that no rebound of the illness follows in the weeks after treatment ends. The patient and her partner should be told that the risk of a puerperal psychosis may approach one in five if there was a previous non-puerperal manic depressive episode. After a previous puerperal psychosis the risk is one in five for a manic illness, and one in 10 for a psychotic depressive illness. For previous schizophrenic or atypical psychosis the risk is less (Platz C, Third International Conference of the Marce Society, Nottingham, 1986).

A patient who conceives while taking lithium and who presents early should stop treatment immediately. If further drug treatment is indicated on clinical grounds neuroleptic drugs or tricyclic antidepressants should be prescribed. A pregnancy which has continued for some time with the mother taking lithium before its discovery is not an automatic indication for termination since the fetal cardiac abnormalities caused by this drug can usually be identified by ultrasound (see previous chapter on identifying abnormalities).

There are some patients whose manic depressive illnesses are so severe or difficult to treat or whose adjustment is so precarious that after the first trimester they will need to continue treatment with lithium, or other neuroleptic maintenance treatment, for the rest of the pregnancy. The serum lithium concentration should be maintained at a value as little above 0·5 mmol/l at 12 hours after ingestion as possible. The daily lithium intake may need to be increased because of the change in the mother's lithium clearance. In these circumstances it is important that contact is established between the doctor monitoring treatment with lithium and other psychotropic drugs and the obstetrician. Obstetric management is easier if the mother is withdrawn gradually from her treatment in the weeks immediately before the estimated date of delivery.

Most puerperal psychoses start soon after delivery, and as withdrawal symptoms do not occur in neonates better protection is conferred by continuing lithium.

A patient still receiving lithium treatment at term should be told to stop taking her tablets as soon as labour starts. No further lithium should be taken during labour and fluid and electrolyte balance must be maintained. The serum lithium concentration must be monitored frequently, and diuretics should be avoided as they will delay lithium excretion.

Ideally, no patient should take benzodiazepines for more than five or six weeks. Some potential mothers take benzodiazepines regularly, however, and they should be offered help with benzodiazepine withdrawal before conception takes place. Public awareness of the possible effects of drugs on pregnancy and the fetus is increasing, but there is little point in inducing guilt and anxiety, which may put the mother in an impossible predicament. Women who have stopped taking benzodiazepines and who are having to cope with the additional pressures of pregnancy will need extra support or even specific psychological treatment. This could be found in a self help group or given individually by a community psychiatric nurse or health visitor.

Recent work suggests that many patients maintained on standard doses of depot neuroleptic drugs may do well on considerably lower doses and may need less additional treatment during any relapse.[19] A pregnant patient who is receiving depot neuroleptic drugs may therefore have her regular dose reduced within the limitations of her clinical state. Depot neuroleptics take some time to clear after the last dose, which may have to be six or eight weeks before delivery is due so that the neonate is free from neuroleptic drugs.

Starting treatment in pregnancy

Treatment should not be skimped just because a patient is pregnant. For anxiety, intermittent use of benzodiazepines is preferable for day or night time exposure to retain the impact of the drug's action, to avoid dependence, and to minimise the effect on the fetus. Benzodiazepines with long half lives and active metabolites such as nitrazepam, diazepam, and chlordiazepoxide are best avoided in favour of drugs such as oxazepam. A depressive illness of the endogenous type, with symptoms such as early morning wakening, diurnal variation, anorexia, poor concentration, guilt, and suicidal ideation, may be treated in the normal way with tricyclic antidepressants if it occurs in pregnancy. If the depression fails to respond to drug treatment electroconvulsive therapy may be used without harming the fetus or causing any long term damage. The need for electroconvulsive therapy seldom occurs, but suicide in the context of a depressive illness in pregnancy is not unknown, and depressive illness at this time demands vigorous action. If treatment is not undertaken problems are likely to occur in the puerperium and afterwards.

Starting treatment in the puerperium

When a mother has suffered a previous episode of psychosis, whether in the puerperium or at another time, both she and her medical attendants will be concerned about the risk of recurrence. As the risk is about 20%, and the interruption to mothering is so profound and long lasting, it is reasonable to offer such mothers prophylactic drug treatment immediately after delivery. Such a decision should be taken jointly by the general practitioner, obstetrician, and psychiatrist. The woman and her partner need to be fully informed and will want assurances about the effect that treatment will have on her, her ability to look after the child, and her ability to breast feed. If the previous episode was a schizophrenic or depressive one treatment with neuroleptic drugs or tricyclic antidepressants is straightforward and is compatible with breast feeding. Unless there is some guidance on dosage from the treatment of a previous episode, it may be necessary to start with small doses and to work up to chlorpromazine 150 mg a day or its equivalent. For tricyclic antidepressants the dose would be that required in treating an endogenous depressive illness in a young adult—that is, between 100 and 150 mg amitriptyline or its equivalent a day. There is no reason to expect any untoward effects on an infant who is breast fed but the health visitor has an important role in monitoring the child's progress.

In a patient with a history of bipolar manic depressive illness lithium is normally the drug of choice; and breast feeding would be contraindicated. Serum concentrations of lithium should be monitored frequently to allow them to reach a full therapeutic value as soon as possible. Most postpartum psychiatric disorders occur within the first four or six weeks. If the mother seems normal at the end of this period the drug can be gradually withdrawn over the next month or two. If, on the other hand, there have been signs of a modified illness treatment should be continued, using the same criteria for continuing treatment as in episodes not occurring in the puerperium. The development of an illness (albeit modified by prophylactic treatment) should be noted because it will have a bearing on the management of that particular patient after any subsequent pregnancy. Should the drug treatment fail to resolve the symptoms further lines of treatment, including electroconvulsive treatment, should be used on the same basis as at any other time. A mother needs to be in as good a position as possible to care for her child, to maintain her marriage, and to have a satisfactory quality of life; the potential for suicide or infanticide in an untreated or partially treated psychotic mother adds emphasis to this point.

1 Kumar R, Robson K. Neurotic disturbance during pregnancy and the puerperium. In: Sandler M, ed. *Mental illness in pregnancy and the puerperium.* Oxford: Oxford University Press, 1979.
2 Cox JL. Psychiatric morbidity and pregnancy: a controlled study of 263 semi rural Ugandan women. *Br J Psychiatry* 1979;309:1282-5.
3 Cox JL, Connor Y, Kendell RE. Prospective study of the psychiatric disorders of childbirth. *Br J Psychiatry* 1982;140:111-7.
3a Kendell RE, Chalmers JC, Platz C. The epidemiology of puerperal psychosis. *Br J Psychiatry* (in press).
4 Rosenberg L., Mitchell AA, Parsella JL, Pashayan H, Louik C, Shapiro S. Lack of relation of oral clefts to diazepam use during pregnancy. *N Engl J Med* 1983;309:1282-5.
5 Kanto JH. The use of benzodiazepines during pregnancy, labour and lactation with particular reference to pharmacokinetic considerations. *Drugs* 1982;23:354-80.
6 Rementeria JL, Bhatt K. Withdrawal symptoms in neonates from intrauterine exposure to diazepam. *Pediatr Pharmacol* 1977;90:123-6.
7 Tomson G, Lunell NO, Sundwall A, Rane A. Transplacental passage and kinetics in the mother and newborn of oxazepam given during labour. *Clin Pharmacol Ther* 1979;25:74-81.
8 Rieder RD. The offspring of schizophrenics—fetal and neonatal deaths. *Arch Gen Psychiatry* 1975;32:200-11.
9 Brockington IF, Kumar R. *Motherhood and mental illness.* London: Academic Press, 1982:249.
10 Edlund MJ, Craig TJ. Antipsychotic drug use and birth defects: an epidemiologic assessment. *Compr Psychiatry* 1984;25:32-7.
11 Hill RM, Desmond MM, Kay JI. Extrapyramidal dysfunction in an infant of a schizophrenic mother. *J Pediatr* 1966;69:589-95.
12 Crombie DL, Pinsent RJ, Fleming D. Imipramine in pregnancy. *Br Med J* 1972;i.802.
13 Webster PA. Withdrawal symptoms in neonates associated with material antidepressant therapy. *Lancet* 1973;ii:318-9.   •
14 Kris EB, Carmichael DM. Chlorpromazine maintenance therapy during pregnancy and confinement. *Psychiatric Quarterly* 1957;31:690-5.
15 Takyi BE. Excretion of drugs in human milk. *Am J Hosp Pharm* 1970;28:317-26.
16 Kallen B, Tandberg A. Lithium and pregnancy—a cohort study on manic depressive women. *Acta Psychiatr Scand* 1983;68:134-9.
17 Ananth J. Side effects in the neonate from psychotropic drugs excreted through breast feeding. *Am J Psychiatry* 1978;135:801-5.
18 Schon M, Amdisen A. Lithium and pregnancy. III. Lithium ingestion by children breast fed by women on lithium treatment. *Br Med J* 1973;ii:138.
19 Manchanda R, Hirsch S. Low dose maintenance medication for schizophrenia. *Br Med J* 1986;293:515-6.

Further reading

Krauer B, Krauer F, Hytten F. *Drug prescribing in pregnancy.* Edinburgh: Churchill-Livingstone, 1984.

Treatment of rheumatic diseases

M A BYRON

Musculoskeletal disorders are common, and conditions such as low back pain and carpal tunnel syndrome may require treatment during pregnancy. Rheumatic conditions are more common in women, with the peak prevalence of rheumatoid arthritis and systemic lupus erythematosus occurring in women of childbearing age. Antirheumatic drugs are, therefore, often required for women of childbearing age.[1]

Table I lists the groups of drugs prescribed for rheumatic conditions. Analgesics and non-steroidal anti-inflammatory drugs are most commonly prescribed, some of which—for example, ibuprofen—are now available without prescription. Several reviews discuss the effects of these drugs during pregnancy and lactation[2-4]

TABLE I—*Antirheumatic drugs*

Drug group	Condition treated
Analgesics Non-steroidal anti-inflammatory drugs	Soft tissue lesions Inflammatory arthritides Osteoarthritis
Antimalarial drugs	Systemic lupus erythematosus Rheumatoid arthritis
Sulphasalazine	Rheumatoid arthritis Ankylosing spondylitis
Gold salts Penicillamine	Severe, persistent rheumatoid arthritis Psoriatic arthritis
Corticosteroids	Systemic lupus erythematosus Rheumatoid arthritis (infrequently) Other connective tissue diseases
Cytotoxic agents	Systemic lupus erythematosus Severe unremitting rheumatoid arthritis Other connective tissue diseases

Non-steroidal anti-inflammatory drugs

Teratogenicity

Studies in animals have linked a variety of skeletal and cranio-vertebral abnormalities with ingestion of large doses of salicylates during pregnancy. In humans several retrospective surveys have shown that significantly more mothers of malformed infants took salicylates regularly during pregnancy than mothers of normal infants.[5] In these studies, however, factors such as the reason for taking salicylates, general health and nutrition of the mothers, and incidence of defects in the families of the malformed children were not always investigated. Three prospective studies have not shown a teratogenic effect of aspirin[6-8] The largest study, the Perinatal Collaborative Project of the United States of America, found that malformation rates were similar in the children of 35 418 women not exposed to aspirin, 9736 with intermediate exposure, and 5128 women heavily exposed during the first four months of pregnancy.[8] Even in women identified as habitual aspirin users the prevalence of congenital malformation was not significantly increased.[7] Overall, therefore, the evidence suggests that salicylates used in recommended doses are unlikely to produce fetal malformations.

Indomethacin is associated with teratogenicity in animals, but the link with human malformation is tenuous.[26] Sulindac, diflunisal, and piroxicam have not been found to be teratogenic in animals, whereas azapropazone and diclofenac have, though at doses greater than those used in humans.[2 9 10] No information is available for the fenamates and tolmetin. Studies in animals have found no evidence of teratogenicity with the commonly prescribed propionic acid derivatives such as ketoprofen, ibuprofen, flurbiprofen, and naproxen.[9]

Effects on fetal growth

A survey from Sydney showed that long term ingestion of aspirin was associated with an increased incidence of stillbirth and reduced birth weight compared with that of controls.[7] Most of the aspirin preparations ingested, however, were compounds containing substances such as phenacetin and caffeine and were taken in large doses. Data from the United States showed no significant effect of aspirin ingestion on birth weight or perinatal mortality.[11] There is no convincing evidence that indomethacin or other non-steroidal anti-inflammatory agents affect fetal growth.

Effects mediated through inhibition of prostaglandin synthesis

Table II summarises the conditions associated with the use of inhibitors of prostaglandin synthesis in pregnancy.

A retrospective study of women with musculoskeletal disorders showed that those who took more than 3·25 g of aspirin a day during the last six months of pregnancy had a significantly longer gestation, longer labour, and greater blood loss at delivery than women who had not taken aspirin.[12] Collins and Turner also found an increased incidence of anaemia, antepartum haemorrhage, and pre-eclampsia in women who took aspirin for long periods.[5] Haemostatic abnormalities and a higher incidence of intracranial haemorrhage have been found in neonates whose mothers ingested aspirin within a few days of delivery.[13 14]

In the fetus prostaglandin E_1 causes relaxation of systemic and pulmonary vessels as well as the ductus arteriosus, and 90% of blood ejected by the right ventricle passes through the ductus arteriosus to the descending aorta.[15] Administration of single doses of an anti-inflammatory agent to a variety of animals results in reversible constriction of the ductus arteriosus and a substantial increase in pulmonary artery pressure in the fetus. Long term exposure to anti-inflammatory agents in animals and humans is

TABLE II—*Conditions associated with use of inhibitors of prostaglandin synthesis in pregnancy*

Effects on mother
    Prolongation of pregnancy
    Prolongation of labour
    Increased blood loss both before and after birth
    Anaemia
    Pre-eclamptic toxaemia

Effects on fetus and neonate
    Haemostatic abnormalities
    Increased incidence of intracranial haemorrhage
    Premature closure of ductus arteriosus
    Persistent pulmonary hypertension

associated with increased amounts of pulmonary artery smooth muscle which results in persistent pulmonary hypertension in the newborn infant, with or without premature closure of the ductus arteriosus.[16] Neonatal respiratory complications attributed to the use of non-steroidal anti-inflammatory drugs in the treatment of premature labour support this association.[7][18] Since other studies, however, have found no increase in fetal mortality when premature labour was suppressed with non-steroid anti-inflammatory drugs,[19] it is likely that the dose and duration of administration of the drug, the gestational age of the fetus at the time of exposure, and the time between the last dose of the drug and the birth of the infant are important factors. Infants born to mothers receiving long term anti-inflammatory treatment are probably most at risk.

Breast feeding

Because non-steroidal anti-inflammatory drugs are weak acids they do not achieve high concentrations in milk. All manufacturers state in their drug information that these drugs should not be used in lactating women. This caution is based on lack of specific information rather than known adverse reactions, and the benefit associated with breast feeding may outweigh the risks of a carefully chosen drug. The appropriate drugs should have a short elimination half life and metabolites which are inert or rapidly eliminated, or both. Hydroxy or methyl metabolites are relatively stable in the infant's stomach whereas glucuronide derivatives may be cleaved, releasing active metabolites.[3] Table III shows the suitability of various drugs. Reported side effects are uncommon, but plasma salicylate concentrations of 24 mg/dl were found in a breast fed child with metabolic acidosis whose mother was taking 2·4 g aspirin a day, and a grand mal fit occurred in a child whose mother was taking indomethacin.[3]

Antimalarial drugs

Chloroquine salts (4-aminoquinolone compounds) cross the placenta and rapidly accumulate in the fetal uveal tract of mice.[20] Teratogenic effects of these substances are probably dose related, and experience from countries where malaria is endemic affirms

TABLE III—*Antirheumatic drug treatment and lactation*

Drugs suitable for use during lactation	Reasons for suitability
Non-steroidal anti-inflammatory drugs	
Ibuprofen	
Flurbiprofen	Small quantities found in milk
Diclofenac	Short elimination half life
Mefenamic acid	Inert metabolites
Sulphasalazine	
Corticosteroids	see text
Drugs not suitable for use during lactation	**Reasons for unsuitability**
Non-steroidal anti-inflammatory drugs	
Salicylates	
Fenoprofen	Glucuronide metabolites
Ketoprofen	
Naproxen	
Piroxicam	
Diflunisal	
Flufenamic acid	Long half life
Tolmetin-Na	
Azapropazone	
Fenbufen	
Sulindac	Active metabolites
Indomethacin	Variable half life; enterohepatic circulation of metabolites
Antimalarial drugs	Risk of retinal damage
Gold salts	
Penicillamine	Potential renal and bone marrow toxicity

the safety of weekly prophylactic doses in pregnancy.[21] Exposure during the first trimester to the doses required to treat rheumatic diseases, however, has resulted in fetal sensorineural hearing loss.[22]

Breast feeding

Both chloroquine and hydroxychloroquine have been found in small quantities in human milk. Despite their widespread use by lactating women for malaria prophylaxis and the lack of reported adverse effects in breast fed infants, the daily doses required for treatment of chronic rheumatic diseases may cause retinal damage, which is difficult to monitor in children of this age. Their use in lactating women is, therefore, not recommended.

Sulphasalazine

Sulphasalazine is increasingly used as a second line treatment in rheumatoid arthritis. Experience with sulphasalazine in the treatment of inflammatory bowel disease has shown that it is safe to use throughout pregnancy and lactation.[4] As it impairs absorption of folic acid, supplementation is recommended during pregnancy.

Gold salts

Both gold thiomalate and auranofin, an oral gold preparation, have proved teratogenic in animals. Gold has been found in the liver and kidneys of an aborted human fetus, and there are reports of possible teratogenic effects.[23][24] Two studies, however, report the safe use of gold during pregnancy,[25][26] and therapeutic gold concentrations have been detected in cord blood without evidence of congenital defects.[27]

Breast feeding

Trace amounts of aurothioglucose have been detected in the milk of lactating women, and gold has been found bound to the red blood cells of breast fed infants.[3] The theoretical possibility of toxicity precludes its use during breast feeding.

Penicillamine

The chelating agent penicillamine (dimethylcysteine) is used for treating Wilson's disease, cystinuria, and rheumatoid arthritis. Its use in pregnancy has been associated with the development of a generalised connective tissue defect, similar to that of Ehlers-Danlos syndrome, in three babies.[28-30] Two died, but in the third the cutis laxa was reversible. Many normal children, however, have been born to mothers taking penicillamine for Wilson's disease,[31][32] and it was proposed that in this disease the fetus was protected from the effects of penicillamine by the excessive maternal pool of copper. In another survey, however, one ventricular septal defect was the only abnormality reported in 27 pregnancies in patients with rheumatoid arthritis and cystinuria.[33]

Breast feeding

Penicillamine is extensively protein bound and has a short half life, so only small amounts should be present in breast milk. No specific investigations in lactation have, however, been carried out. The potential toxicity makes its use hazardous.

Corticosteroids

The pharmacology of corticosteroids and potential effects on the fetus are discussed in the chapter on treatment of asthma. In two studies of pregnancy associated with corticosteroid treatment 37 pregnancies in 24 patients with rheumatic diseases were evaluated.[34][35] Although five pregnancies resulted in abortion and four in fetal death, this was in a group of patients at high risk of fetal loss. Length of gestation and birth weight were within normal limits and a few minor fetal abnormalities were considered unrelated to steroid treatment in the mother. Both studies emphasised the importance of giving the mother additional corticosteroids during delivery and the rarity of fetal adrenocortical insufficiency.

Breast feeding

In the doses most commonly used for treating rheumatic diseases (15 mg of prednisone a day or less) there is little chance of an infant receiving appreciable amounts of prednisolone in breast milk.[36]

Cytotoxic drugs

Alkylating agents and antimetabolites may be teratogenic and mutagenic, and even if used after the first trimester of pregnancy the fetus is susceptible to bone marrow depression, infection, and haemorrhage.[37] Azathioprine is the cytotoxic agent most commonly used in rheumatic disorders. In a study of 125 pregnancies in renal transplant recipients taking both azathioprine and prednisone only one infant showed a congenital abnormality, though a number had lymphopenia, growth retardation, and an increase in chromosomal breakage.[38] Results of long term follow up studies in these children are not available. The risk of lymphoproliferative and gonadal disorders would be likely to cause concern.

Breast feeding

Many cytotoxic drugs are found in appreciable amounts in human milk, and the risk to the infant would outweigh any benefits of breast feeding.

Guidelines for antirheumatic treatment in pregnancy

Adequate explanations of the possible risks of any proposed treatment, with appropriate advice on contraception, are essential when treating women of childbearing age. The use of drugs that pose the least threat to the fetus will minimise anxiety should pregnancy occur. In women with established rheumatic diseases it is important to appreciate that without the use of agents which suppress the disease pregnancy may not have occurred or may not have been carried to term. Adequate control of the disease may also enable a woman to feel capable of bearing and raising children. There is a good chance of remission of rheumatoid arthritis during pregnancy, though aggressive treatment may continue to be necesary in systemic lupus erythematosus.[2]

Non-steroidal anti-inflammatory agents

Drug action is a function of concentration and time. To minimise the effects on the fetus drugs with a short elimination half life and inactive metabolites—for example, ibuprofen, flurbiprofen, and ketoprofen—should be used at the maximum tolerated dosage interval. The most potent inhibitors of prostaglandin synthesis, such as salicylates and indomethacin, should be avoided throughout pregnancy, if possible, and certainly during the last trimester. Well motivated women with moderate symptoms may be managed with simple analgesics, paracetamol being the drug of choice.

Drugs that modify rheumatic disease

Only a small proportion of women require disease modifying drugs. Antimalarial drugs are contraindicated in pregnancy or lactation, whereas sulphasalazine appears to be safe, though folate supplements should be given. Treatment with gold and penicilla-

65

mine should not be started during pregnancy, and these drugs should not be used by breast feeding women. If a woman becomes pregnant while taking these drugs gold can be continued at the longest possible dosage interval and penicillamine should be slowly reduced or withdrawn. Pyroxidine supplements are recommended as penicillamine may deplete maternal stores.[3] Careful consideration should be given to the use of cytotoxic agents in pregnancy. Although azathioprine appears to be relatively safe, long term follow up data are not yet available. Corticosteroids in the doses required to treat rheumatic conditions seem to be safe in pregnancy and lactation. Additional doses are needed to cover delivery. Fetal adrenal insufficiency is rare.

1 Hill RM. Drugs ingested by pregnant women. *Clin Pharmacol Ther* 1973;**14**:654–9.
2 Needs CJ, Brooks PM. Antirheumatic medication in pregnancy. *Br J Rheumatol* 1985;**24**:282–90.
3 Needs CJ, Brooks PM. Antirheumatic medication during lactation. *Br J Rheumatol* 1985;**24**:291–7.
4 de Swiet M, ed. *Medical disorders in obstetric practice*. Oxford: Blackwell Scientific, 1984.
5 Collins E. Maternal and fetal effects of acetaminophen and salicylates in pregnancy. *Obstet Gynecol* 1981;**58**:(suppl 5):57–62.
6 Buckfield P, Major congenital faults in newborn infants: a pilot study in New Zealand. *N Z Med J* 1973;**78**:195–204.
7 Turner G, Collins E. Fetal effects of regular salicylate ingestion in pregnancy. *Lancet* 1975;ii:338–40.
8 Slone D, Heinonen O, Kaufman DW, Siskind V, Monson RR, Shapiro S. Aspirin and congenital malformations. *Lancet* 1976;i:1373–5.
9 Anti-rheumatic drugs. In: Huskisson EC, ed. *Clinics in rheumatic diseases*. London: W B Saunders, 1979;5:2.
10 Anti-rheumatic drugs II. In: Huskisson EC, ed. *Clinics in rheumatic diseases*. London: W B Saunders, 1980;6:3.
11 Shapiro S, Monson RR, Kaufman DW, Siskind V, Heinonen O, Slone D. Perinatal mortality and birth weight in relation to aspirin taken during pregnancy. *Lancet* 1976;i:1375–6.
12 Lewis RB, Shulman JD. Influence of acetylsalicylic acid, an inhibitor of prostaglandin synthesis, on the duration of human gestation and labour. *Lancet* 1973;ii:1159–61.
13 Rumack CM, Guggenheim MA, Rumack BH, Peterson RG, Johnson ML, Braithwaite WR. Neonatal intracranial hemorrhage and maternal use of aspirin. *Obstet Gynecol* 1981;**58**(Suppl 5):52–6.
14 Stuart MJ, Gross SJ, Elrad H, Graeber JE. Effects of acetylsalicylic-acid ingestion on maternal and neonatal hemostasis. *N Engl J Med* 1982;**307**:909–12.
15 Rudolph AM. The effects of non-steroidal anti-inflammatory compounds on fetal circulation and pulmonary function. *Obstet Gynecol* 1981;**58**(Suppl 5):63–7.
16 Levin DL, Mills LJ, Weinberg AG. Haemodynamic pulmonary vasculature and myocardial abnormalities secondary to pharmacologic constriction of fetus ductus arteriosus: a possible mechanism for persistent pulmonary hypertension and transient tricuspid insufficiency in the new born infant. *Circulation* 1979;**60**:360–4.
17 Zuckerman H, Reiss V, Rubenstein I. Inhibition of human premature labour by indomethacin. *Obstet Gynecol* 1974;**44**:787–9.
18 Wilkinson AR, Aynsley-Green A, Mitchell MD. Persistent pulmonary hypertension and abnormal prostaglandin E levels in preterm infants after maternal treatment with naproxen. *Arch Dis Child* 1979;**54**:942–5.

19 Wiquist N, Lundstrom V, Green K. Premature labour and indomethacin. *Prostaglandins* 1975;**10**:515–26.
20 Ullberg S, Lindquist N, Sjostrand S. Accumulation of chorio-retinotoxic drugs in the foetal eye. *Nature* 1970;**227**:1257–8.
21 Lewis R, Lauersen NH, Birnbaum S. Malaria associated with pregnancy. *Obstet Gynecol* 1973;**42**:696–700.
22 Hart CW, Naunton RF. The ototoxicity of chloroquine phosphate. *Arch Otolaryngol* 1964;**80**:407–12.
23 Rocker I, Henderson WJ. Transfer of gold from mother to fetus. *Lancet* 1976;**ii**:1246.
24 Rogers JG, Anderson RMcD, Chow CW. Possible teratogenic effects of gold. *Aust Paediatr J* 1980;**16**:195–8.
25 Stern L. Drug therapy in the perinatal period. In: Morselli PL, Garattini S, Sereni S, eds. *Basic and therapeutic aspects of perinatal pharmacology*. New York: Raven Press, 1975:7–12.
26 Zvaifler NJ. Gold and anti-malarial therapy. In: McCarty DJ, ed. *Arthritis and allied conditions*. 9th ed. Philadelphia: Lea and Febiger, 1979:357.
27 Cohen DL, Orzd J, Taylor A. Infants of mothers receiving gold therapy. *Arthritis Rheum* 1981;**24**:104–5.
28 Mjolnerod OK, Dommerud SA, Rasmussen K, Gjeruldsen ST. Congenital connective tissue defect probably due to d-penicillamine treatment in pregnancy. *Lancet* 1971;**i**:673–5.
29 Solomon L. Abrams G, Dinner M, Berman L. Neonatal abnormalities associated with d-penicillamine treatment during pregnancy. *N Engl J Med* 1977;**296**:54–5.
30 Linares A, Zarranz JJ, Rodriguez-Alarcon J, Diaz-Perez JL. Reversible cutis laxa due to maternal d-penicillamine therapy. *Lancet* 1979;**ii**:43.
31 Scheinberg IH, Sternlieb I. Pregnancy in penicillamine treated patients with Wilson's disease. *N Engl J Med* 1975;**293**:1300–2.
32 Walshe JM. Pregnancy in Wilson's disease. *Q J Med* 1977;**46**:73–83.
33 Lyle WH. Penicillamine in pregnancy. *Lancet* 1978;**i**:606–7.
34 Popert AJ. Pregnancy and adreno cortical hormones, some aspects of their interactions in rheumatic diseases. *Br Med J* 1962;**i**:967–72.
35 Yackel DB, Kempers RD, McConahey WM. Adrenocorticosteroid therapy in pregnancy. *Am J Obstet Gynecol* 1966;**96**:985–9.
36 McKenzie SA, Selley JA, Agnew JE. Secretion of prednisolone into breast milk. *Arch Dis Child* 1975;**50**:894–6.
37 Barber HRK. Fetal and neonatal effects of cytotoxic agents. *Obstet Gynecol* 1981;**58**:Suppl 5):41–7.
38 Nolan GH, Sweet RL, Laros RK. Renal cadaver transplantation followed by successful pregnancies. *Obstet Gynecol* 1974;**4**:732–9.

Treatment of endocrine diseases

W M HAGUE

This chapter reviews the use of drugs in pregnancy in all the main endocrine disorders with the exception of diabetes mellitus, which is dealt with separately in this book and in an excellent review by Vaughan and Oakley.[1]

Drugs are used in both diagnosis and management of endocrine diseases. Diagnosis entails assessing basal function of an endocrine gland followed by tests to suppress or stimulate the gland. Further diagnostic measures may well include procedures to localise a lesion. Medical management usually takes the form of hormone replacement treatment in the case of endocrine failure or suppressive treatment in the case of hyperfunction.

Diagnosis

Pregnancy usually requires a state of endocrine balance—that is, the chances of conceiving are reduced unless the endocrine milieu is normal. Endocrine disease does, however, arise de novo in both pregnancy and the puerperium. This section deals with the appropriate tests which require the use of drugs.

Thyrotoxicosis—After diabetes, thyrotoxicosis is the most common endocrine disorder developing in pregnancy, many of the signs mimicking those of normal pregnancy. Until recently diagnosis of borderline cases would have used the thyrotrophin releasing hormone test to assess pituitary thyrotrophin (thyroid stimulating hormone) response. Doubts have been expressed about the use of thyrotrophin releasing hormone in early pregnancy because it produces smooth muscle contraction.[2] The sensitive radioimmunometric assay for thyroid stimulating hormone has virtually replaced the thyrotrophin releasing hormone test, at least in pregnancy. Other diagnostic measures in thyrotoxicosis include measurement of iodine-131 uptake, a test which is totally contra-indicated in pregnancy because of the risk of fetal uptake of the isotope and subsequent damage to the thyroid, although complete destruction of the thyroid has not been documented with the diagnostic dose.[3]

Other less common conditions that may present in pregnancy are the adrenal disorders which cause hypertension.

Phaeochromocytoma may be suspected with increased excretion of catecholamines or their metabolites. Pentolinium, a quarternary ammonium ganglion blocking compound, has been used as a diagnostic agent. Failure to reduce plasma catecholamine concentrations after intravenous injection of 5 mg pentolinium provides additional evidence for establishing the diagnosis,[4] but no experience of this test in pregnancy has been described. Localisation procedures for phaeochromocytoma include the use of ^{131}I-met-iodobenzylguanidine, but this should be avoided in pregnancy because of the radiation risk to the fetal thyroid.

Conn's syndrome—Mineralocorticoid excess, which occurs in Conn's syndrome, is rare but may be suspected in patients with hypertension and hypokalaemia. The hypertension is rarely severe and full investigation may be postponed until after pregnancy, when localisation procedures such as the use of radio labelled selenium cholesterol may be used without fear of affecting the fetus.

Cushing's syndrome—Though rare, glucocorticoid excess presenting in pregnancy is much more serious, and needs urgent investigation because of the high risk (16%) of malignancy of the adrenal cortex.[5] Dexamethasone crosses the placenta, causing suppression of the fetal pituitary-adrenal axis,[6] but in the doses used for disgnosis this suppression is short lived. The use of metyrapone is discussed in the section on management.

Pituitary disorders—Investigation of pituitary disorders usually includes assessing the response to insulin induced by hypoglycaemia. The transient nature of the hypoglycaemia is without serious risk to the fetus. The usual precautions of having an intravenous line open, with hydrocortisone and dextrose drawn up ready, as well as using a smaller dose of insulin for patients with suspected hypopituitarism, apply in pregnancy as much as for non-pregnant patients.

Management: hormone replacement treatment

Hypothyroidism

Hypothyroidism is usually diagnosed and treated before pregnancy as the hypothyroid state is associated with infertility. Patients with untreated hypothyroidism have a high risk of spontaneous abortions, a stillbirth rate twice that in normal pregnancies, and an increased incidence of premature labour and subnormal neonatal neurological development in their children.[3] An increased risk of congenital abnormality in the children of these patients has been refuted.[7] Thyroid replacement is achieved with thyroxine 100–200 µg/day as a single dose; the response is monitored by the fall in the serum concentration of thyroid stimulating hormone. Thyroxine requirements do not change in pregnancy; the dose can usually be maintained despite the oestrogen mediated rise in thyroxine binding globulin that occurs in normal pregnancy.[8] The important point is to monitor and treat patients according to biochemical findings rather than by clinical judgment. If the dose of thyroxine has been increased during pregnancy it will need to be reduced in the puerperium. There is no contraindication to breast feeding.

Hypoadrenalism

As with hypothyroidism, adrenal insufficiency is usually diagnosed and treated before pregnancy. Replacement treatment (hydrocortisone 20–30 mg/day, fludrocortisone 0·05–0·20 mg/day) is essential and does not need to be changed in pregnancy unless intercurrent stress or illness develops, when increased or parenteral doses should be given. The oestrogen mediated rise in cortisol binding globulin during pregnancy does not seem to affect steroid requirements. There is one report of an increased incidence of infants who were small for gestational age in patients with Addison's disease, but it is not clear whether this was due to the disease or the treatment.[9] No other complications, either fetal or maternal, associated with steroid replacement treatment have been reported. There is no contraindication to breast feeding.

Hypopituitarism

Anterior pituitary deficiency states require thyroxine and corticosteroid replacement treatment as described above, with the exception that fludrocortisone is not required since mineralocorticoid secretion is independent of the pituitary. Untreated, hypopituitarism has a high mortality for both fetus and mother.[10] Hypogonadotrophic states may require exogenous gonadotrophin or, more physiologically, pulsatile gonadotrophin releasing hormone treatment to achieve ovulation. Once pregnancy is achieved, however, maintenance treatment is not necessary because gonadotrophin and sex steroids are produced by the fetoplacental unit. Lactation may be impaired because of protein deficiency.

Posterior pituitary failure is associated with diabetes insipidus and requires replacement treatment with the vasopressin analogue desmopressin (5–10 µg twice daily). A review of 67 cases showed that 58% of patients deteriorated during pregnancy.[11] The mechanism for this is unclear but may reflect the increase in glomerular filtration rate in pregnancy. No ill effects of desmopressin in pregnancy have been reported apart from the small risk of increased uterine contractility owing to its oxytocin like structure and activity.[12] This effect, however, is seen when desmopressin is used intravenously as a diagnostic agent rather than with the normal replacement regimen using nasal insufflation. The oxytocic action of desmopressin is only a fraction ($^1/_{75}$) of that of arginine vasopressin.

Hypoparathyroidism

Hypoparathyroidism usually occurs as a complication in patients who have undergone thyroidectomy, but occasionally it is seen as part of an autoimmune condition or as a hormone resistant syndrome. Hypoparathyroidism in the mother poses severe risks of fetal hyperparathyroidism with neonatal hypocalcaemic rickets, which may be fatal. Treatment with calcium (1600–2000 µg/day) and either vitamin D (1·25–2·5 mg/day) or dihydrotachysterol (250–1000 µg/day) is essential, and maternal serum calcium and phosphate values should be monitored regularly to maintain normocalcaemia.[13] Vitamin D requirement increases twofold to threefold during pregnancy.[14] The use of calcitriol has been associated

71

with fetal hypermineralisation in one of twin fetuses.[14] In the puerperium the requirement for calcium and vitamin D should be reassessed; they may not be required at all.[15] In healthy women an insignificant amount of vitamin D is secreted in the breast milk,[16] but the high doses of vitamin D required in lactating hypoparathyroid women may cause neonatal hypervitaminosis.

Ovarian failure

Until recently the prospect of pregnancy in a patient with ovarian failure seemed remote. The development of techniques of embryo transfer, however, has made pregnancy a real possibility for these patients. Preparation of the patient includes the use of oestrogen and progesterone to prepare the recipient uterus and endometrium before embryo transfer and subsequently to maintain the hormonal environment until the fetoplacental unit can take over. The use of sex steroids in pregnancy is discussed below.

Management: endocrine gland hyperfunction

Thyrotoxicosis

The mainstay of medical treatment of thyrotoxicosis is the thionamide agents: carbimazole, propylthiouracil, and, less commonly in the United Kingdom, methimazole. Propylthiouracil is less lipid soluble and more highly protein bound than carbimazole or methimazole, and is less readily transferred into breast milk[17] or, theoretically, across the placenta. No teratogenic effects have been reported for propylthiouracil or carbimazole, but there have been five cases of a scalp defect, aplasia cutis, occurring in neonates whose mothers had been treated with methimazole.[18] One study suggested that maternal thyrotoxicosis may itself be associated with fetal malformation and that the risk may be reduced by antithyroid drug treatment.[19] Perinatal mortality is also high in untreated thyrotoxicosis, with an increased incidence of premature delivery; this can be reduced to normal with treatment.[20] Fetal hypothyroidism is a definite risk with all thionamide treatment, and the lowest possible dose to maintain biochemical euthyroidism in the mother must be used, with (at least) monthly measurements of the serum concentrations of free thyroxine (or free thyroxine index) and thyroid stimulating hormone. Fetal goitre formation may occur but is not dose related, being also affected by the antibody status and iodine intake of the mother.[8] The intellectual development of children exposed to antithyroid drugs in utero is reported to be unaffected.[21] Autoimmune thyrotoxicosis often improves during pregnancy so that the dosage may be reduced. After delivery, however, sudden overactivity is common, requiring an increase in treatment.[22]

Other agents used to control thyrotoxicosis include β blocking drugs, potassium iodide, and radioactive iodine. β blocking drugs are discussed in full in the chapter on cardiovascular disease. Potassium iodide, which is often used in preparation for thyroid surgery, is well recognised as a cause of fetal goitre.[8] Cases of fetal goitre have been reported when the mother took as little as 12 mg iodide a day. Radioactive iodine (^{131}I) in therapeutic doses is liable to ablate the fetal thyroid and also has the potential to induce maternal thyroid storm. Oddly, the risk to the fetus is least in the first trimester before the fetal iodine trap is operational.[23]

In the light of the above, propylthiouracil is probably the drug of choice in both pregnancy and puerperium. Initially 100–150 mg should be taken every 8 hours, and this should be reduced to 50 mg every 6–8 hours once the hyperthyroid state is controlled clinically and, more importantly, biochemically. The lowest possible maintenance dose should be used to maintain the serum free thyroxine concentration in the high normal range. If thyrotoxicosis recurs or is not controlled up to 600 mg/day in divided doses may be used.[20] Failure to control symptoms may indicate the need for partial thyroidectomy, in which case propranolol 40 mg may be given every 6 hours to control residual symptoms and reduce vascularity before the operation.[8]

Fetal and neonatal thyrotoxicosis may occur as a result of transplacental passage of thyroid stimulating antibodies in the absence of maternal signs after thyroid ablation or, rarely, in maternal autoimmune hypothyroidism. Fetal thyrotoxicosis has been successfully treated with thionamide using the fetal heart rate as a guide to dosage.[24] Intra-amniotic administration of thyroxine has been used in a case of suspected fetal hypothyroidism,[25] but experience with this is limited and careful screening and follow up of such infants is needed.

Cushing's syndrome

Drugs used in the management of Cushing's syndrome include metyrapone and trilostane. Both of these drugs block various points in the biosynthetic pathway of cortisol. Experience of their use in pregnancy is limited because of the rarity of the syndrome. Both agents cross the placenta and affect fetal and placental steroid metabolism. Metyrapone has not been shown to have any adverse effects on the fetus or mother in normal pregnancy,[26] but its effect on urinary oestrogen excretion is uncertain.[5] Studies in baboons have shown an inhibition of surfactant release, although the infants did not develop respiratory distress.[27] Trilostane, which antagonises 3βOH-steroid dehydrogenase, inhibits placental progesterone production with the risk of abortion or premature labour[28]; it is therefore contraindicated in pregnancy. Metyrapone has been used successfully in a pregnant woman with Cushing's syndrome with survival of both mother and infant.[5] In another case, however, the use of metyrapone coincided with the onset of severe pre-eclampsia at just over 26 weeks' gestation, and the baby died as a result of a complication of premature delivery.[29] The link between the use of metyrapone, which increases 11-deoxycorticosterone production, and the exacerbation of maternal hypertension in this case is not clear.

In view of the high incidence (16%) of adrenal malignancy among pregnant patients with Cushing's syndrome, active surgical or obstetric management, or both, has been recommended in the first and last trimesters; metyrapone should be reserved for difficult cases in the second trimester.[30] Metyrapone is lipid soluble and is therefore likely to be excreted into the breast milk; there are no data on its use by lactating women.

Congenital adrenal hyperplasia

Adrenal suppression in patients with congenital adrenal hyperplasia is achieved with replacement glucocorticoid and mineralocorticoid treatment, which should be maintained in pregnancy as for patients with hypoadrenalism (see above). In a recent study treatment of a fetus with adrenal hyperplasia was achieved by giving dexamethasone to the mother in the first and second trimesters to suppress fetal production of adrenocorticotrophic hormone, thus reducing fetal adrenal androgen output with its associated masculinisation of female genitalia.[31]

Phaeochromocytoma

Surgical treatment is required for phaeochromocytoma in pregnancy once the effects of circulating catecholamines have been controlled by α and β adrenoceptor blocking agents.

Hyperprolactinaemia and acromegaly

The dopaminergic agent bromocriptine is the drug of choice in the management of hyperprolactinaemia caused by pituitary microadenoma or macroadenoma, allowing ovulation to occur and reducing tumour size. Bromocriptine may be used in the management of acromegaly as it reduces growth hormone secretion, but treatment is not always successful. It is also used to suppress lactation. No adverse effects on the fetus have been reported, either in women in whom ovulation was induced with bromocriptine or in women given bromocriptine throughout pregnancy,[32] although there is evidence that bromocriptine, or an active metabolite, crosses the placenta.[33]

Treatment with bromocriptine in pregnancy should be reserved for the small number of women who present with symptoms and signs of tumour expansion in whom a high resolution computed tomography scan confirms the diagnosis and in whom immediate delivery is not practicable or desirable. Treatment starts at 5 mg/day in divided doses, doubling daily over three days until symptoms resolve or the patient is taking 20 mg/day or has developed side effects. An operation is rarely necessary. Lactation in such patients is both suppressed and contraindicated, and early contraception must be considered after delivery.

Hyperparathyroidism

Surgical treatment is required for symptomatic hyperparathyroidism in pregnancy. Fluid replacement may be necessary before the operation if the hypercalcaemia is severe.[34] The neonate needs careful observation for signs of hypocalcaemia (secondary to parathormone suppression), which may present late in the postnatal period.

Sex hormones and pregnancy

Compounds which contain oestrogen are commonly used to inhibit ovulation and thus avoid pregnancy. In practice, pregnancy has often occurred during oestrogen treatment because of impaired absorption, a missed pill, or too low a dose. In the past oestrogens were also used to inhibit lactation. Non-steroidal oestrogens, such as stilboestrol, hexoestrol, and dienoestrol, are teratogenic and have a well documented association with adenocarcinoma of the vagina and cervix in the daughters of mothers who took these drugs before the 18th week of gestation.[35] Other changes of the female genital tract have been shown, and testicular, seminal, and other genital abnormalities have been found in the sons of such mothers.[36]

Steroidal oestrogens do not have the same effects as the stilboestrol like compounds,[35] but there is disagreement about their teratogenicity. Anomalies of the cardiovascular system, limb deformities, neural tube defects, and renal and tracheo-oesophageal abnormalities have all been attributed to steroidal oestrogens.[37] Two large prospective studies, however, have not found any increased risk to babies born to mothers who conceived either after or while taking oral contraceptives.[38 39]

Many of the progestogens used as contraceptive agents, such as norethisterone and levonorgestrel, are 19-nortestosterone derivatives with mildly androgenic properties and could therefore cause virilisation of a female fetus. The small amounts present in oral contraceptives, however, are unlikely to do so. On the other hand, 17-hydroxyprogesterone derivatives, such as medroxyprogesterone acetate (Provera) and 17-hydroxyprogesterone caproate (Proluton), are pure progestational compounds and may have a role in the management of habitual abortion and premature labour, although their use remains controversial.[3]

The weak androgen danazol has been used in the treatment of endometriosis to suppress ovarian activity and menstruation. Ovulation does occasionally occur at low doses, and danazol treatment has been associated with masculinisation of a female fetus.[40] Concurrent non-hormonal contraception should be used.

The antiandrogen cyproterone acetate has been shown to inhibit masculinisation of the male fetus in studies in animals[41] and should be given with oestrogen to provide contraception as well as to enhance the antiandrogenic effects. No such effects have been reported in the fetuses of women taking small amounts of cyproterone acetate such as those found in Diane. The antioestrogen clomiphene citrate has been implicated in several case reports of neural tube defects. Large studies, however, have not shown any significant increase in the malformation rate.[42] The use of sex steroids by lactating women deserves comment. Administration of high doses of oestrogen to suppress lactation, for a long time considered a risk because of thromboembolism,[43] is now absolutely contraindicated, and bromocriptine should be used instead. On the other hand, the use of low dose ($\leqslant 50\ \mu g$) oestrogen compounds for contraception is unlikely to inhibit lactation.[16] Because the risk of venous thromboembolism is greatest post partum, however, it is wise to avoid compounds containing oestrogen in the immediate and early puerperium. Progestogen only contraception may be preferable as it has no effect on lactation or coagulation.[44] If milk supply is diminishing or needs supplementation, or when menses return, transfer to a combined preparation is recommended if maximum contraceptive effectiveness is required. Cyproterone acetate is contraindicated until weaning is complete as it may be transferred into the breast milk,[45] although its effects on the neonate are unknown.

1 Vaughan NJA, Oakley NW. Treatment of diabetes in pregnancy. *Clin Obstet Gynaecol* 1986;**13**:291–306.
2 Reynolds JEF, ed. *Martindale; the extra pharmacopoeia*. London: Pharmaceutical Press, 1982:1276–7.
3 Hays PM, Cruikshank DP. Hormonal therapy during pregnancy. In: Eskes TKAB, Finster M, eds. *Drug therapy during pregnancy*. London: Butterworths, 1985:110–60.
4 Brown MJ, Allison DJ, Jenner DA, Lewis PJ, Dollery CT. Increased sensitivity and accuracy of phaeochromocytoma diagnosis achieved by use of plasma-adrenaline estimation and a pentolinium-suppression test. *Lancet* 1981;i:174–7.
5 Gormley MJJ, Hadden DR, Kennedy TL, Montgomery DAD, Murnaghan GA, Sheridan B. Cushing's syndrome in pregnancy—treatment with metyrapone. *Clin Endocrinol* 1982;**16**:283–93.
6 Funkhouser JD, Peery KJ, Mockridge PB, Hughes ER. Distribution of dexamethasone between mother and fetus after maternal administration. *Pediatr Res* 1978;**12**:1053–6.
7 Echt DR, Doss JF. Myxedema in pregnancy. Report of 3 cases. *Obstet Gynecol* 1963;**22**:615–20.
8 Burr W. Thyroid disease. *Clin Gynaecol* 1986;**13**:277–90.
9 Osler M. Addison's disease and pregnancy. *Acta Endocrinol* 1962;**41**:67–78.
10 Grimes HG, Brooks MH. Pregnancy in Sheehan's syndrome. Report of a case and review. *Obstet Gynecol Surv* 1980;**35**:481–8.

11 Hime MC, Richardson JA. Diabetes insipidus and pregnancy. Case report, incidence, and review of the literature. *Obstet Gynecol Surv* 1978;**33**:35–9.
12 van der Wilt B, Drayer JIM, Eskes TKAB. Diabetes insipidus in pregnancy as a first sign of a craniopharyngioma. *Eur J Obstet Gynaecol Reprod Biol* 1980;**10**:269–74.
13 Montoro M, Mestman JH. How to manage parathyroid disease in the pregnant patient and neonate. *Contemporary Obstetrics and Gynaecology* 1981;**17**:143–57.
14 Salle BL, Berthezene F, Glorieux FH, et al. Hypoparathyroidism during pregnancy: treatment with calcitriol. *J Clin Endocrinol Metab* 1981;**52**:810–3.
15 Wright AD, Joplin GF, Dixon HG. Post-partum hypercalcaemia in treated hypoparathyroidism. *Br Med J* 1969;i:23–5.
16 Beeley L. Drugs and breastfeeding. *Clin Obstet Gynaecol* 1986;**13**:247–51.
17 Kampmann JP, Hansen JM, Johansen K, Helweg J. Propylthiouracil in human milk. *Lancet* 1980;i:736–7.
18 Mujtaba Q, Burrow GN. Treatment of hyperthyroidism in pregnancy with propylthiouracil and methimazole. *Obstet Gynecol* 1975;**46**:282–6.
19 Momotani M, Ito K, Hamada N, Ban Y, Nishikawa Y, Mimura T. Maternal hypothyroidism and congenital malformation in the offspring. *Clin Endocrinol* 1984;**20**:695–700.
20 Burrow GN. Thyroid diseases. In: Burrow GN, Ferris TF, eds. *Medical complications during pregnancy*. Philadelphia: W B Saunders, 1982:187–214.
21 Burrow GN, Bartsocas D, Klatskin DH, Grunt JA. Children exposed in utero to propylthiouracil. *Am J Dis Child* 1968;**116**:161–5.
22 Amino N, Miyai K, Yamamoto T, et al. Transient recurrence of hyperthyroidism after delivery in Graves' disease. *J Clin Endocrinol Metab* 1977;**44**:130–6.
23 Stouffer SS, Hamburger JT. Inadvertent ^{131}I therapy for hypothyroidism in the first trimester of pregnancy. *J Nucl Med* 1976;**17**:146–9.
24 Cove DH, Johnston P. Fetal hypothyroidism: experience of treatment in four siblings. *Lancet* 1985;i:430–2.
25 Lightner ES, Fismer DA, Giles H, Woolfenden J. Intra-amniotic injection of thyroxine (T_4) to a human fetus. *Am J Obstet Gynecol* 1977;**127**:487–90.
26 Heinen G, Buchheit M, Oertal W. Untersuchungen mit dem adrenostatikum SU4885 (Metopiron) in der schwangerschaft. *Klin Wochensch* 1963;**41**:103–5.
27 Kling OR, Kotas RV. Endocrine influences on pulmonary maturation and the lecithin/sphingomyelin ratio in the fetal baboon. *Am J Obstet Gynecol* 1975;**12**:664–8.
28 van der Spuy ZM, Jones DL, Wright CSW, et al. Inhibition of 3β hydroxysteroid dehydrogenase activity in first trimester human pregnancy with trilostane and WIN 32729. *Clin Endocrinol* 1983;**19**:521–32.
29 Connell JMC, Cordiner J, Davies DL, Fraser R, Frier BM, McPherson SG. Pregnancy complicated by Cushing's syndrome: potential hazard of metyrapone therapy. Case report. *Br J Obstet Gynaecol* 1985;**92**:1192–5.
30 van der Spuy ZM, Jacobs HS. Management of endocrine disorders in pregnancy—part II. *Postgrad Med J* 1984;**60**:312–20.
31 David M, Forest MG. Prenatal treatment of congenital adrenal hyperplasia resulting from 21-hydroxylase deficiency. *J Pediatr* 1984;**105**:799–803.
32 Krupp P, Turkalj I. Bromocryptine safety monitoring in pregnancy. In: Jacobs HS, ed. *Prolactinomas and pregnancy*. Lancaster: MTP Press, 1984:45–50.
33 Bigazzi M, Ronga R, Lancranjan I, et al. A pregnancy in an acromegalic woman during bromocryptine treatment: effects on growth hormone and prolactin in the maternal, fetal and amniotic compartments. *J Clin Endocrinol Metab* 1979;**48**:9–12.
34 Clark D, Seeds JW, Cefalo RC. Hyperparathyroid crisis and pregnancy. *Am J Obstet Gynecol* 1981;**140**:840–2.
35 Herbst AL, Kurman RJ, Scully RE, Poskanzer DC. Clear-cell adenocarcinoma of the genital tract in young females: registry report. *N Engl J Med* 1972;**287**:1259–64.
36 Stillman RJ. In utero exposure to diethylstilboestrol: adverse effects on the reproductive tract and reproductive performance in male and female offspring. *Am J Obstet Gynecol* 1982;**142**:905–21.
37 Wilson JG, Brent RL. Are female sex hormones teratogenic? *Am J Obstet Gynecol* 1981;**141**:567–80.
38 Royal College of General Practitioners' Oral Contraception Study. The outcome of pregnancy in former oral contraceptive users. *Br J Obstet Gynaecol* 1976;**83**:608–16.

39 Vessey M, Meisler L, Flavel R, Yeates D. Outcome of pregnancy in women using different methods of contraception. *Br J Obstet Gynaecol* 1979;**86**:548–57.
40 Shaw RW, Farquhar JW. Female pseudohermaphroditism associated with danazol exposure in utero. Case report. *Br J Obstet Gynaecol* 1984;**91**:386–9.
41 Hamada H, Neumann F, Junkmann K. Intrauterine antimaskuline Beeinflussung von Rattenfeten durch ein stark gestagen wirksames Steroid. *Acta Endocrinol* 1963;**44**:380–8.
42 Kurachi K, Aono T, Minigawa J, Miyake A. Congenital malformations of newborn infants after clomiphene-induced ovulation. *Fertil Steril* 1983;**40**:187–9.
43 Daniel DG, Campbell H, Turnbull AC. Puerperal thromboembolism and suppression of lactation. *Lancet* 1967;ii:287–9.
44 Guillebaud J. Combined oral contraceptive pills, In: London N, ed. *Handbook of family planning*. Edinburgh: Churchill Livingstone, 1985:53–98.
45 Stoppelli I, Rainer E, Humpel M. Transfer of cyproterone acetate to the milk of lactating women. *Contraception* 1980;**22**:485–93.

Treatment of cardiovascular diseases

KENNEDY R LEES, PETER C RUBIN

Drugs required in pregnancy for cardiovascular disorders fall into two major categories: antiarrhythmic and antihypertensive agents. Antihypertensive agents have been widely used, and both controlled and uncontrolled trials have been performed with these drugs in pregnancy. Experience of their use in the first trimester is limited, however, so the absence of reports of malformation cannot be equated with safety. The rarity of cardiac arrhythmias during pregnancy means that most information is anecdotal or retrospective. Further information on the use of drugs for cardiovascular disorders during pregnancy is contained in recent detailed reviews.[1-6]

Antiarrhythmic drugs

The indications for starting antiarrhythmic treatment in pregnancy are the same as in non-obstetric practice. Most experience has been gained with digoxin, quinidine, and the β blockers.

Digoxin

There have been no reports of digoxin causing malformation. Digoxin crosses the human placenta, and toxic maternal concentrations can be fatal to the fetus. At therapeutic concentrations, however, digoxin does not appear to have an adverse effect on the fetus. There is some evidence that digoxin increases myometrial tone,[7] resulting in shorter pregnancy and labour.[8] Digoxin is found in human breast milk in concentrations similar to those in maternal serum. Thus the daily dose to a breast fed infant may be about 1–2 µg; one report showed no detectable digoxin in the infant's blood during breast feeding.[9] Digoxin is safe to use throughout pregnancy and the puerperium provided that maternal serum concentrations do not rise above the therapeutic range. Digoxin clearance by the kidney increases during pregnancy. If the dosage remains unchanged, by the end of pregnancy the serum concentration will have fallen to about half the value before pregnancy. It is therefore important to measure the digoxin concentration at intervals during and after pregnancy.

Digoxin is the drug of choice for control of atrial fibrillation, atrial flutter, and paroxysmal supraventricular tachycardia in pregnancy. Like all antiarrhythmic drugs it is indicated as a prophylactic agent only when the arrhythmia to be treated has been shown to be recurrent, sustained, and poorly tolerated.

Quinidine

Teratogenesis has not been reported with quinidine. At therapeutic concentrations it appears to be safe, and the drug has only mild oxytocic activity.[10] Some quinidine is found in human breast milk but at concentrations below those of maternal plasma. Quinidine is normally 80% protein bound. Changes in plasma protein concentrations during pregnancy cause total plasma quinidine concentrations to fall and free concentrations to be underestimated. This must be taken into account when interpreting drug monitoring data. After delivery total concentrations of quinidine increase by half.

Quinidine is the drug of choice for the treatment during pregnancy of premature extrasystoles, Wolff-Parkinson-White syndrome, and ventricular arrhythmias and for treatment after cardioversion of supraventricular tachycardia.

Procainamide

Procainamide has not been associated with teratogenesis. The drug crosses the placenta but does not appear to have any adverse effects. In view of the association with the lupus syndrome procainamide should be reserved for patients who failed to respond to quinidine.

Lignocaine

There is no evidence to suggest that lignocaine is teratogenic.

Later in pregnancy moderate doses over short periods appear to be safe. Fetal blood concentrations are about half of the maternal values, and the fetus is capable of metabolising lignocaine by term. The use of lignocaine in the presence of fetal hypoxia may be dangerous, however, since ion trapping may cause concentration of lignocaine in the fetal circulation. No information is available on the effects of pregnancy on lignocaine disposition.

Disopyramide

Disopyramide has not yet been widely studied in pregnancy. It crosses the placenta, resulting in fetal concentrations which are about 40% of the maternal values, and is also found in breast milk. One report suggested that it may cause uterine contractions.[11] Experience with this drug in pregnancy is too limited to draw conclusions about the effect of pregnancy on its disposition.

Verapamil

There is little experience in the use of verapamil in pregnancy. One group reported no teratogenic or adverse effects in pregnancy.[12] It is known to cross the placenta, resulting in fetal concentrations about 40% of maternal values. The effects of pregnancy on verapamil disposition have not been described.

In summary, present experience is greatest with digoxin, quinidine, and lignocaine. Most arrhythmias occurring in pregnancy may be treated by one of these three drugs.

Antihypertensive drugs

Although the risks of maternal hypertension during pregnancy are clearly recognised, the benefits to the fetus of pharmacological intervention remain controversial. Results of controlled studies suggest that treatment of both chronic hypertension and pregnancy induced hypertension is beneficial to the fetus, but the size of these studies limits the ability to draw definitive conclusions.[13 14] Redman *et al* studied 247 women with chronic hypertension and reported nine miscarriages or perinatal deaths in their control group and only one in the treated group.[13] In a study of women who developed hypertension during pregnancy Rubin *et al* showed a reduction in both maternal blood pressure and neonatal morbidity in the treatment group compared with the control group.[14] Recommendations about the level of blood pressure which warrants treatment during pregnancy are controversial, particularly since blood pressure is normally expected to fall to a nadir in the mid-trimester. Our own, admittedly aggressive, policy is to treat chronic hypertension at a pressure above 140/90 mm Hg after the first trimester and to treat hypertension which develops during pregnancy if there has been a rise of 30 mm Hg systolic or 15 mm Hg diastolic above the values before pregnancy or during the first trimester.

First line agents in mild to moderate hypertension

Methyldopa has been used for many years in pregnancy, but there have been no reports of serious adverse effects on the fetus. It crosses the placenta and is found in the amniotic fluid. The largest reported study showed no adverse effect on the fetus,[13] and follow up studies of the children for over seven years have confirmed the safety of the drug.[15] When given near term methyldopa was associated with a reduction in systolic blood pressure in neonates, but their stress response was normal.[16]

Methyldopa is effective in controlling chronic hypertension during pregnancy. It does not, however, reduce the incidence of superimposed pre-eclampsia. Although unwanted side effects (sedation, depression, and postural hypotension) may necessitate discontinuation of the drug in about 15% of women, its good safety record makes methyldopa the drug of choice in treating chronic hypertension in pregnancy.

β Blockers—There is no evidence of a teratogenic effect of β blockers. There have been a few reports of fetal abnormality, but these must be viewed in the light of the background incidence of deformities.

Several studies have assessed the effects of β blockers later in pregnancy. All of these drugs cross the placenta, producing fetal concentrations similar to those in maternal plasma. There was initially some concern that propranolol might inhibit fetal growth, but subsequent studies suggest that growth is at most only slightly retarded.[14 17-21] Some reports have implicated propranolol in the reduction of fetal heart rate variability, an effect not confirmed with atenolol. Various β blockers have been linked with serious neonatal morbidity, particularly hypotension and hypoglycaemia. These anecdotal observations have not been confirmed by placebo controlled prospective trials with atenolol[14] or metoprolol,[22] however, and almost certainly reflect the complications of the disease rather than the actions of the drugs.

All of the β blockers are found in breast milk in varying concentrations, but the dose to the neonate is clinically insignificant. Pregnancy has no clinically important effects on the disposition of β blockers.

Good blood pressure control has been achieved with metoprolol, oxprenolol, labetalol, atenolol, acebutolol, and propranolol in both chronic hypertension and pregnancy induced hypertension. There is little to choose between the various β blockers.

Both β blockers and methyldopa are effective antihypertensive agents. Comparative studies have shown little difference between them in the outcome of pregnancy.[17 23–25] A β blocker may be better tolerated by the mother, but methyldopa has the advantage of a reassuring long term follow up for the infant.

Second line agents in moderate to severe hypertension

Hydralazine has not been widely used in the first trimester. Blood pressure is lowered without any reduction in uteroplacental blood flow.[26]

It is known to cross the placenta, but the only recorded problem in neonates exposed to hydralazine during late pregnancy has been occasional thrombocytopenia,[27] which may take up to three weeks to reverse. Only low concentrations of hydralazine are found in breast milk. It is not known whether pregnancy alters the disposition of hydralazine.

Except in the acute management of hypertensive emergencies, when it is given parenterally, hydralazine should be given as second line treatment to poorly controlled patients after failure to respond to methyldopa or a β blocker.

Prazosin—There have been no reports of teratogenesis with prazosin, and the available evidence suggests that it is safe later in pregnancy. Satisfactory control of blood pressure and fetal growth were recorded in 25 patients with pregnancy induced hypertension treated with prazosin combined with oxprenolol.[28] Small doses are usually sufficient.

Diuretics are widely used in non-obstetric practice for controlling hypertension and treating cardiac failure. The use of loop diuretics in pregnancy for treatment of cardiac failure appears to be safe, and a recent review of the use of thiazides for the control of hypertension in pregnancy concluded that there was no evidence of a deleterious effect.[4] Nevertheless, pre-eclampsia is a condition in which intravascular volume depletion occurs, and further depletion by diuretics may have a critical effect on the compromised uteroplacental blood flow. For this theoretical reason diuretics are not generally used for controlling hypertension during pregnancy.

Drugs for hypertensive emergencies

Diazoxide—There are no reports on the use of diazoxide in the first trimester. It crosses the placenta and has been implicated in abnormal hair growth and development.[29] Prolonged exposure late in pregnancy is commonly associated with neonatal hyperglycaemia. Diazoxide is not well cleared by the neonate.[29]

Early experience with diazoxide was based on the misguided belief that rapid infusion of large boluses was required. Subsequent experience shows that the risk of severe maternal hypotension is diminished or abolished when lower doses (30–100 mg) are given more slowly. The hypotensive effect is obtained without altering uterine blood flow.[30] Diazoxide should be reserved for use in intrapartum emergencies.

Sodium nitroprusside—There is little published information on the use of this drug in pregnancy. Short term use has been satisfactory in small numbers of patients. When facilities exist for accurate and continuous blood pressure monitoring sodium nitroprusside is the drug of choice for treating hypertensive emergencies and eclampsia.

1 Rubin PC. Treatment of hypertension in pregnancy. *Clin Obstet Gynaecol* 1986;13:1–11.
2 Rotmensch HH, Elkayam O, Frishman W. Antiarrhythmic drug therapy during pregnancy. *Ann Intern Med* 1983;98:487–97.
3 Lubbe WF. Hypertension in pregnancy: pathophysiology and management. *Drugs* 1984;28:170–88.
4 Collins R, Yusof S, Peto R. Overview of randomised trials of diuretics in pregnancy. *Br Med J* 1985;290:17–23.
5 Berkowitz RL. Anti-hypertensive drugs in the pregnant patient. *Obstet Gynecol Surv* 1980;35:191–204.

6 Rubin PC. Beta-blockers in pregnancy. *N Engl J Med* 1981;305:1323–6.

7 Norris PR. The action of cardiac glycosides on the human uterus. *Journal of Obstetrics and Gynaecology of the British Commonwealth* 1961;68:916–29.

8 Weaver JB, Pearson JK. Influence of digitalis on time of onset and duration of labour in women with cardiac disease. *Br Med J* 1973;ii:519–20.

9 Loughman PM. Digoxin excretion in human breast milk. *J Pediatr* 1978;92:1019–20.

10 Ueland K, McAnulty JH, Ureland FR, Metcalfe J. Special considerations in the use of cardiovascular drugs. *Clin Obstet Gynaecol* 1981;24:809–23.

11 Leonard RF, Brown TE, Levy AM. Initiation of uterine contractions by disopyramide during pregnancy. *N Engl J Med* 1978;299:84–5.

12 Barrilon A, Grand A, Gerbaux A. Treatment of the heart during pregnancy. *Ann Med Interne* (Paris) 1974;125:437–45.

13 Redman CWG, Beilin LJ, Bonnar J, Ounsted MK. Fetal outcome in trial of antihypertensive treatment in pregnancy. *Lancet* 1976;ii:753–6.

14 Rubin PC, Butters L, Clark DM, et al. Placebo-controlled trial of atenolol in treatment of pregnancy-associated hypertension. *Lancet* 1983;i:431–4.

15 Cockburn J, Moar VA, Ounsted M, Redman CWG. Final report of study on hypertension during pregnancy: the effects of specific treatment on the growth and development of the children. *Lancet* 1982;i:647–9.

16 Whitelaw A. Maternal methyldopa treatment and neonatal blood pressure. *Br Med J* 1981;283:471.

17 Gallery EDM, Saunders DM, Hunyor SN, Gyory AZ. Randomised comparison of methyldopa and oxprenolol for treatment of hypertension in pregnancy. *Br Med J* 1979;i:1591–4.

18 Oakley GDG, McGarry K, Limb DG, Oakley CM. Management of pregnancy in patients with hypertrophic cardiomyopathy. *Br Med J* 1979;i:1749–50.

19 Eliahou HE, Silverberg DS, Reisin E, Romem I, Mashiachs, Serr DM. Propranolol for the treatment of hypertension in pregnancy. *Br J Obstet Gynaecol* 1978;85:431–6.

20 Tcherdakoff PH, Colliard M, Berrard E, Kreft C, Dupay A, Bernaille JM. Propranolol in hypertension during pregnancy. *Br Med J* 1978;ii:670.

21 Boh-Kanner G, Schweitzer A, Reisner SH, Joel-Cohen SJ, Rosenfeld JB. Propranolol and hydralazine in the management of essential hypertension in pregnancy. *Br J Obstet Gynaecol* 1980;87:110–4.

22 Wichman K. Hypertension in pregnancy—a methodological study and a double blind study of the effects of metoprolol in the mother, fetus and neonate. Linkoping, Sweden: Linkoping University, 1986. (Dissertation No 217.)

23 Williams ER, Morrisey JR. A comparison of acebutolol with methyldopa in the hypertensive pregnancy. *Pharmatherapeutica* 1983;3:487–91.

24 Fidler J, Smith B, Fayers P, de Swiet M. Randomised controlled comparative study of methyldopa and oxprenolol in treatment of hypertension in pregnancy. *Br Med J* 1983;286:1927–30.

25 Livingstone I, Craswell PW, Bevan EB, Smith MT, Eadie MJ. Propranolol in pregnancy. A three year prospective study. *Clin Exp Hypertens* 1983;B2:341–50.

26 Lunell, NO, Lewander R, Nylund L, Sarby B, Thornstrom S. Acute effect of dihydralazine on uteroplacental blood flow in hypertension during pregnancy. *Gynecol Obstet Invest* 1983;16:274–82.

27 Widerlov E, Karlman I, Storsater J. Hydralazine-induced neonatal thrombocytopenia. *N Engl J Med* 1980;303:1235.

28 Lubbe WF, Hodge JV. Combined alpha- and beta-adrenoreceptor antagonism with prazosin and oxprenolol in control of severe hypertension in pregnancy. *NZ Med J* 1981;691:169–72.

29 Milner RDG, Chouksey SK. Effects of fetal exposure to diazoxide in man. *Arch Dis Child* 1972;47:537–43.

30 Caritis S, Morishima HO, Stark RI, James LS. The effect of diazoxide on uterine blood flow in pregnant sheep. *Obstet Gynecol* 1976;48:464–8.

Anticoagulants

M DE SWIET

The main indications for the use of anticoagulants in pregnancy are the treatment and prevention of deep vein thrombosis and pulmonary embolus and the anticoagulation treatment of patients with artificial heart valves. The increased risk of thromboembolism and the vulnerability of the fetus to oral anticoagulants make management of anticoagulant treatment in pregnancy particularly difficult.

Safety of anticoagulants during pregnancy

Heparin

There is no evidence that heparin is teratogenic; it does not cross the placenta. A retrospective review of published work suggested that the incidence of fetal loss may be as high with heparin as with warfarin (see below),[1] but this has not been confirmed in a small clinical trial.[2] There may, however, be a slightly increased risk of premature labour.[2] Heparin is probably not secreted in breast milk, but, even if it were, it would be inactivated in the infant's stomach.

The main problems associated with heparin are bleeding and bone demineralisation in the mother. Bleeding usually occurs because of excess heparin administration, which is rare in patients taking subcutaneous heparin in doses up to 20 000 units a day in pregnancy or 16 000 units a day after delivery. Since heparin is excreted by the kidney, patients who have renal insufficiency or pre-eclampsia are at extra risk. Patients should not bleed because of excess heparin administration, even at delivery or during surgical procedures, if the heparin assay is less than 0·4 units/ml.[3]

More intensive intravenous heparin treatment, such as that used in the first phase of treatment of deep vein thrombosis, is associated with a high risk of bleeding, particularly if the heparin is given intermittently rather than by continuous infusion. If the protamine sulphate neutralisation test shows a concentration of heparin greater than 1 unit/ml there is a definite risk of spontaneous bleeding.[4] Patients may also bleed because of thrombocytopenia induced by heparin treatment.[5-7] This is an uncommon idiosyncratic reaction related to the formation of platelet antibodies.

Maternal bone demineralisation was also considered an idiosyncratic reaction as a few patients taking 10 000 units of heparin a day or more for at least three months have suffered crushed vertebrae and rib fractures.[8-10] It appears, however, that subclinical bone demineralisation may occur in a large proportion of women taking heparin for three months or more. The mechanism is unknown, although reduced concentrations of 1, 25-dihydroxy vitamin D have been implicated.[12]

Warfarin

Warfarin is teratogenic. It causes abnormalities of cartilage and bones, chondrodysplasia punctata,[13] and, rarely, the asplenia syndrome.[14] Although these are definite risks, the incidence of such abnormalities is probably less than 5% in women taking warfarin in the first trimester. For example, none occurred in 22 pregnancies during which women with artificial heart valves took warfarin in the first trimester.[15] There is also a high abortion rate associated with warfarin,[15] but it is not clear to what extent the condition for which the warfarin is being used contributes to this risk.[16] In addition, warfarin has been associated with abnormalities of the central nervous system such as microcephaly, optic atrophy, cranial nerve palsies, and hydrocephalus.[17] These abnormalities are not specific to treatment at any particular stage of the pregnancy. Since warfarin crosses the placenta freely, it has been suggested that they are due to repeated small episodes of intracerebral haemorrhage. Such haemorrhage is even more likely to occur at the end of pregnancy and during labour, when frank intracerebral and retroplacental haemorrhages have been reported.[18] Warfarin is not secreted in breast milk in appreciable amounts.[19]

The risk of bleeding in the mother is not specific to pregnancy, but women may bleed for other reasons in pregnancy, and warfarin certainly exacerbates this risk. Secondary postpartum haemorrhage and wound haematomas are major risks in women taking warfarin in the first 10 days after delivery.[20]

Phenindione

It has been claimed that some of the adverse fetal effects associated with warfarin are less common in patients taking phenindione, but there is inadequate clinical experience to confirm this.[21] In contrast to warfarin phenindione is excreted in breast milk and this has caused bleeding in the neonate.[22]

Thrombolytic treatment

Streptokinase and urokinase have both been used in pregnancy,[23] but they have not been studied recently. Such drugs may cause bleeding, premature labour,[24] and incoordinate uterine action, which may be due to release of fibrin degradation products.[25]

Effect of pregnancy on clinical efficacy of anticoagulants

Heparin

Because the concentrations of clotting factors increase in pregnancy higher doses of heparin—that is, 10 000 units 12 hourly—are prescribed for subcutaneous prophylactic treatment. It is not known exactly when concentrations of these clotting factors return to normal after delivery, but blood volume also decreases after delivery and therefore the dose of heparin is usually decreased to 8000 units 12 hourly or 5000 units eight hourly.

Warfarin

Warfarin requirements probably do not change during pregnancy. In the few cases in which warfarin is prescribed in pregnancy, however, there will be concern about its effects on the fetus. These may be dose related, so warfarin dosage is usually adjusted to maintain a prothrombin ratio at the lower, rather than the higher, end of the therapeutic range (1·8–4).

Clinical use of anticoagulants during pregnancy

Pulmonary embolus and deep vein thrombosis

Because of the unreliability of clinical diagnosis and the risks of anticoagulant treatment every effort should be made to make the diagnosis of pulmonary embolus objectively, even in pregnancy.[26] Patients with pulmonary embolus who remain shocked one hour after the initial episode should be treated by pulmonary embolectomy. If this is not available thrombolytic treatment should be considered. The place of surgical treatment in the management of massive iliofemoral thrombosis is unclear. All other patients should be treated with anticoagulants.

Initial treatment should be with intravenous heparin given by continuous infusion, starting at a dose of 40 000 units a day (1600 units an hour). Patients with large thromboses may require higher infusion rates. Although the partial thromboplastin time is often used for control of heparin treatment, we have found that the protamine sulphate neutralisation test is more helpful clinically.[4] This test measures the concentration of heparin in the blood, which should be 0·6 to 1·0 units/ml. After an arbitrary period of five to ten days, subcutaneous heparin should be substituted. Warfarin should not be used in these cases because of the risks to the fetus. The initial dose of subcutaneous heparin is 10 000 units 12 hourly. This is a low dose which does not affect the whole blood clotting time or the partial thromboplastin time. The dose is controlled by the heparin assay,[27] which should be less than 0·4 units/ml. The heparin assay should be repeated as often as the patient would normally attend the clinic for antenatal care. Patients can give themselves the heparin and may be discharged from hospital. The only inconveniences are pain at the injection site and bruising. Because of the continuing risk of recurrent thromboembolism subcutaneous heparin treatment should be continued for the remainder of pregnancy and through labour, provided that the heparin assay is less than 0·4 units/ml. Epidural anaesthesia should not be given because of the small risk of epidural haematoma.[28]

After delivery the dose of heparin must be reduced to 8000 units 12 hourly. The length of time after delivery that anticoagulants should be continued is unknown; six weeks is generally recommended.[29] One week after delivery, when the risk of secondary postpartum haemorrhage has diminished, treatment may be changed to warfarin if the patient prefers oral treatment. Since warfarin treatment necessitates frequent prothrombin estimation warfarin is initially not much less inconvenient than heparin for the patient. As stated above, breast feeding is safe for women taking heparin or warfarin[19] but not phenindione.

Prophylaxis against venous thromboembolism

What prophylaxis, if any, should be used in a pregnant woman who has had deep vein thrombosis or a pulmonary embolus in the past? The risk of recurrence in pregnancy appears to be 5%[30] to 13%[31] irrespective of the circumstances of the previous episode of thromboembolism and its nature. Drugs which have been shown by clinical trial to reduce the risk of thromboembolism associated with surgery (not in pregnancy) include dextran, warfarin, and heparin. It is clearly impractical to use dextran throughout pregnancy, and warfarin should not be used for routine prophylaxis for the reasons indicated above.

The question remains whether subcutaneous heparin should be used throughout pregnancy. In a patient who has had a single episode of thromboembolism heparin should probably not be used because of the risks of heparin treatment indicated above and, in particular, because of the risk of bone demineralisation, which has occurred in patients taking as little as 10 000 units of heparin a day.[10] If this form of bone demineralisation is similar to osteoporosis it will be resistant to treatment and exacerbated by the menopause. Treatment with lower doses of heparin (less then 10 000 units a day), other heparinoids,[32] or heparin with vitamin D and calcium supplementation may obviate the risks of conventional prophylactic heparin treatment and also be effective. Until these suggestions have been tested by clinical trial, however, prophylactic heparin treatment is not justified in the antenatal period in patients who have had a single episode of thromboembolism in the past.

Our policy with such patients is to counsel them about the varied clinical presentation of thromboembolism in the antenatal period and to urge them to attend hospital if they have any warning symptoms; to use specific prophylaxis in the antenatal period; and to give them 1 litre of dextran 70 over about six hours in labour, thus permitting epidural anaesthesia. After delivery these patients should be treated with subcutaneous heparin 8000 units every 12 hours for at least one week. This may be changed to warfarin after one week if the patient wishes, but a total of six weeks' treatment should be given after delivery as described above. The major risks with this policy are thromboembolism in the antenatal period and anaphylaxis caused by dextran. We reported one possible antenatal pulmonary embolism in 26 patients treated in this way[30] and have subsequently managed another 20 patients without further thromboembolism. Anaphylaxis should not be a problem provided the first part of the dextran infusion is given slowly. Since dextran may interfere with blood group cross matching, blood samples must be taken for cross matching before giving dextran.

Patients who have the rare antithrombin III, protein C, or protein S deficiencies require special management in pregnancy.[33] Other parents who have had more than one episode of thromboembolism but in whom no predisposing cause can be found should be warned before pregnancy that they are probably at increased risk and offered heparin prophylaxis throughout pregnancy. Patients with lupus anticoagulant are paradoxically also at risk of developing thromboembolism,[34] which may be arterial. It is not clear to what extent treatment with prednisone or aspirin, which have been advocated for the management of this condition in pregnancy,[34 35] reduce this risk. Our practice has been to offer such patients intrapartum and postnatal prophylaxis as described above if they have a history of thromboembolism but to withhold prophylaxis if they have no such history.

Patients with artificial heart valves

Patients with artificial heart valves are usually treated with warfarin. In pregnancy, because of the problems associated with warfarin treatment, attempts have been made to substitute subcutaneous heparin. This is unacceptable, however, because of the catastrophic risks of peripheral arterial embolisation or thrombosis of the valve in situ.[15 36-37] Possible alternative treatments such as subcutaneous heparin and dipyridamole,[38] high dose subcutaneous heparin,[39] or long term intravenous heparin[40] need to be assessed by clinical trial. Until there is adequate satisfactory experience of these alternative treatments such patients should continue to take warfarin in pregnancy despite the risks to both fetus and mother. The patient should be warned about these risks before pregnancy and ideally before the original operations. These risks may, however, have been exaggerated.[41] So far as pregnancy is concerned, there is no doubt that tissue valves, which do not need anticoagulation, are superior to artificial valves.[42] Unfortunately they do not last so long.[43]

Although warfarin is generally recommended for the management of these patients in pregnancy,[44] the risk of fetal and maternal bleeding becomes too great at the end of pregnancy and during delivery. At about 36 weeks' gestation high dose intravenous heparin should be substituted for warfarin and given by continuous infusion to maintain a heparin concentration of 0·6 to 1·0 units/ml. About two weeks' later, by which time the anticoagulant effects of warfarin on the fetus should have worn off, and if the situation is obstetrically favourable, the patient should be delivered. This can be achieved safely by stopping heparin treatment and delivering the patient 6–12 hours later, when the thrombin time has been shown to be normal. After delivery high dose intravenous heparin should be restarted, and this should be changed to warfarin about one week later.

Conclusion

Anticoagulant treatment should not be undertaken lightly in pregnancy. It poses additional risks to both the mother and the fetus. Further clinical trials are necessary to determine the best ways to manage prophylaxis for patients who have had thromboembolism in the past and also for those with artificial heart valves.

1 Hall JG, Pauli RM, Wilson KM. Maternal and fetal sequelae of anticoagulation during pregnancy. *Am J Med* 1980;**68**:122–40.
2 Howell R, Fidler J, Letsky E, de Swiet M. The risk of antenatal subcutaneous heparin prophylaxis: a controlled trial. *Br J Obstet Gynaecol* 1983;**90**:1124–8.
3 Bonnar J. Thromboembolism in obstetric and gynaecological patients. In: Nicolaides AN, ed. *Thromboembolism aetiology, advances in prevention and management*. Lancaster: MTP Press, 1975:311–34.
4 Dacie J. *Practical haematology*. Edinburgh: Churchill Livingstone, 1975:413–4.

5 Cines DB, Kaywin P, Bina M, Tomaski A, Schreiber AD. Heparin-associated thrombocytopenia. *N Engl J Med* 1980;**303**:788–95.
6 Chong BH, Pitney WR, Castaldi PA. Heparin-induced thrombocytopenia: association of thrombotic complications with heparin-dependent IgG antibody that induces thromboxane synthesis and platelet aggregation. *Lancet* 1982;ii:1246–8.
7 Hatjis CG. Heparin-induced thrombocytopenia in pregnancy. *J Repro Med* 1984;**29**:337–8.
8 Griffith GC, Nichols G, Asher JD, Hanagan B. Heparin osteoporosis. *JAMA* 1965;**193**:91–4.
9 Avioli LV. Heparin-induced osteopenia: an appraisal. *Adv Exp Med Biol* 1975;**52**:375–87.
10 Griffiths HT, Liu DTY. Severe heparin osteoporosis in pregnancy. *Postgrad Med J* 1984;**60**:424–5.
11 de Swiet M, Dorrington Ward P, Fidler J, et al. Prolonged heparin therapy in pregnancy causes bone demineralisation (heparin induced-osteopenia). *Br J Obstet Gynecol* 1983;**90**:1129–34.
12 Aarskog D, Lage A, Markestad T, Ulstein M, Sagen N. Heparin-induced inhibition of 1, 25–dihydroxyvitamin D formation. *Am J Obstet Gynecol* 1984;**148**:1141–2.
13 Stevenson RE, Burton M, Ferlauto GJ, Taylor HA. Hazards of oral anticoagulants during pregnancy. *JAMA* 1980;**243**:1549–51.
14 Cox DR, Martin L, Hall BD. Asplenia syndrome after fetal exposure to warfarin. *Lancet* 1977;ii:1134.
15 Chen WWC, Chan CS, Lee PK, Wang RYC, Wong VCW. Pregnancy in patients with prosthetic heart valves: an experience with 45 pregnancies. *Q J Med* 1982;**51**:358–65.
16 Javares T, Coto EC, Maiques V, Rincon A, Such M, Caffarena JM. Pregnancy after heart valve replacement. *Int J Cardiol* 1984;**5**:731–9.
17 Holzgreve W, Cary JC, Hall BD. Warfarin-induces fetal abnormalities. *Lancet* 1976;ii:914–5.
18 Villasanta U. Thromboembolic disease in pregnancy. *Am J Obstet Gynecol* 1965;**93**:142–60.
19 Orme M L'E, Lewis PJ, de Swiet M, et al. May mothers given warfarin breast-feed their infants? *Br Med J* 1977;i:1564–5.
20 de Swiet M, Letsky E, Mellows H. Drug treatment and prophylaxis of thromboembolism in pregnancy. In: Lewis PJ, ed. *Therapeutic problems in pregnancy.* Lancaster: MTP Press, 1977:81–9.
21 Oakley CM, Hawkins DF. Pregnancy in patients with prosthetic heart valves. *Br Med J* 1983;**287**:358.
22 Eckstein H, Jack B. Breast feeding and anticoagulant therapy. *Lancet* 1970;i:672–3.
23 Pfeifer GW. The use of thrombolytic therapy in obstetrics and gynaecology. *Australian Annals of Medicine* 1970;suppl:28–31.
24 Amias AG. Streptokinase, cerebral vascular disease—and triplets. *Br Med J* 1977;i:1414–5.
25 Hall RJC, Young C, Sutton GC, Cambell S. Treatment of acute massive pulmonary embolism by streptokinase during labour and delivery. *Br Med J* 1972;iv:647–9.
26 de Swiet M. Thromboembolism. In: de Swiet M, ed. *Medical disorders in obstetric practice.* Oxford: Blackwell Scientific, 1984:95–115.
27 Denson KWE, Bonnar J. The measurement of heparin: a method based on the potentiation of anti-factor Xa. *Thrombosis et Diathesis Haemorrhagica* 1973;**30**:471.
28 Crawford JS. *Principles and practice of obstetric anaesthesia.* 4th ed. Oxford: Blackwell Scientific, 1978:182–3.
29 de Swiet M, Bulpitt CJ, Lewis PJ. How obstetricians use anticoagulants in the prophylaxis of thromboembolism. *Journal of Obstetrics and Gynaecology,* 1980;**1**:29–32.
30 Lao TT, de Swiet M, Letsky E, Walters BNJ. Prophylaxis of thromboembolism in pregnancy: an alternative. *Br J Obstet Gynaecol* 1985;**92**:202–6.
31 Badaracco MA, Vessey M. Recurrence of venous thromboembolism disease and use of oral contraceptives. *Br Med J* 1974;i:215–7.
32 Harenberg J, Zimmerman R, Schwartz F, Kübler W. Treatment of heparin-induced thrombocytopenia with thrombosis by new heparinoid. *Lancet* 1983;i:986–7.
33 de Swiet M. Thromboembolism. *Clin Haematol* 1985;**14**:643–60.
34 Lubbé WF, Butler WS, Palmer SJ, Liggins GC. Lupus anticoagulant in pregnancy. *Br J Obstet Gynaecol* 1984;**91**:357–63.
35 Ware Branch D, Scott JR, Kochenour NK, Hershgold E. Obstetric complications associated with the lupus anticoagulant. *N Engl J Med* 1985;**13**:1322–6.

36 Bennett GG, Oakley CM. Pregnancy in a patient with a mitral valve prosthesis. *Lancet* 1968;i:616–9.
37 Wang RYC, Lee PK, Chow JSF, Chen WWC. Efficacy of low-dose, subcutaneously administered heparin in treatment of pregnant women with artificial heart valves. *Med J Aust* 1983;2:126–8.
38 Biale Y, Cantor A, Lewen Thal H, Gueron M. The course of pregnancy in patients with artificial heart valves treated with dipyridamole. *International Journal of Obstetrics and Gynaecology* 1980;18:128–32.
39 Rabinovici J, Mani A, Barkai G, Hod II, Frenkel Y, Mashiach S. Long term ambulatory anticoagulation by constant subcutaneous heparin infusion in pregnancy. *Br J Obstet Gynaecol* 1987;94:89–91.
40 Nelson DM, Stempel LE, Fabri PJ, Talbert M. Hickman catheter use in a pregnant patient requiring therapeutic heparin anticoagulation. *Am J Obstet Gynecol* 1984;149:461–2.
41 Chong MKB, Harvey D, de Swiet M. Follow up study of children whose mothers were treated with warfarin during pregnancy. *Br J Obstet Gynaecol* 1984;91:1070–3.
42 Beadle EM, Luepker RV, Williams PP. Pregnancy in a patient with porcine valve xenografts. *Am Heart J* 1979;98:510–2.
43 Kirklin JW. The replacement of cardiac valves. *N Engl J Med* 1981;304:291–2.
44 Oakley CM. Pregnancy in patients with prosthetic heart valves. *Br Med J* 1983;286:1680–2.

Epilepsy and anticonvulsant drugs

ANTHONY HOPKINS

An epileptic seizure is a paroxysmal discharge of cerebral neurones resulting in a clinical event apparent to the subject or an observer, or both. Tonic-clonic (grand mal) seizures are common and most disruptive of life, but many patients have combinations of complex partial (temporal lobe) seizures and tonic-clonic seizures. Epilepsy, which is best defined as a continuing tendency to epileptic seizures, affects about 0·5% of women of childbearing age.[1] Thus family doctors and obstetric units will from time to time have a pregnant woman with epilepsy under their care. A unit delivering 3000 mothers a year will have about 15 pregnant women with epilepsy on their books at any one time.

It must be remembered that seizures, particularly if they occur in the third trimester, may be due to eclampsia rather than epilepsy. Although modern antenatal care makes it unlikely that eclamptic seizures will occur without previous evidence of pre-eclampsia, many patients presenting with eclampsia have not attended for antenatal care. Furthermore, eclampsia may appear suddenly, particularly during or after delivery.

Epilepsy and oral contraception

Some women with epilepsy may become pregnant unexpectedly while taking oral contraceptives if they are also taking phenytoin. This drug induces hepatic hydroxylating enzymes so that the metabolism of phenytoin itself and many steroids, including oestrogens, is increased. Pregnancy is more likely to occur if a low oestrogen contraceptive is used, but women taking pills containing 50 µg of oestrogen may also become pregnant. Women must be advised of this risk and either use an alternative method of contraception or change their anticonvulsant treatment if they do not wish to become pregnant.

First seizures in pregnancy and epilepsy which begins in pregnancy

The age specific annual incidence of epilepsy is roughly constant at 40–50 cases per 100 000 women throughout the childbearing period.[1] In some women pregnancy and the onset of non-eclamptic seizures will therefore coincide by chance. There is no statistical evidence that pregnancy is likely to precipitate epilepsy. Occasionally, non-eclamptic seizures may occur for the first time in pregnancy, remit after delivery, and then return only in subsequent pregnancies.[2] Knight and Rhind found only two such patients among 59 epileptic mothers studied during 153 pregnancies.[2] In women with pre-existing epilepsy it is unusual for seizures to recur during pregnancy after a prolonged period without seizures. The apparent rarity of such events indicates that pregnancy itself is not a particularly potent epileptogenic agent.

A patient who starts to have seizures during pregnancy should be referred to a neurologist, who will decide whether investigation of the cause is necessary. Investigation is essential if neurological signs develop in association with the seizures or if there are other symptoms such as headache. Seizures with a partial onset also require investigation. An electroencephalogram is unlikely to help in diagnosing the cause but may be helpful in deciding the type of seizure and therefore appropriate anticonvulsant treatment. Computed tomography is required for diagnosing a structural lesion. This is reasonably safe for the fetus, which can be protected from scattered radiation by suitable lead curtains and abdominal screening. Magnetic resonance scanning may be an alternative choice.

Although tumours are rare causes of seizures in women of reproductive age,[3] some epileptogenic tumours, such as meningiomas, expand during pregnancy.[4] Arteriovenous malformations may expand or infarct during pregnancy and, late in pregnancy or in the immediate puerperium, seizures may be due to cortical venous thrombosis.[5]

Frequency of seizures during pregnancy

Schmidt reviewed 27 studies of the effect of pregnancy on the course of epilepsy published between 1884 and 1980 and found considerable variation in the frequency of seizures.[6] For example, in one study 75% of patients had more seizures and 8% had fewer; in another study 33% had more seizures and 52% had fewer. The average experience from all the studies listed by Schmidt in a total of 2165 women was an increase in frequency of seizures in 24% and a decrease in 22%; in 53% of women the frequency of seizures remained unchanged. Many of these studies are now out of date since increased knowledge of the changes in metabolism of anticonvulsant drugs during pregnancy has enabled better control of oral dosage and serum concentrations.

Schmidt et al studied the course of 23 pregnancies in women who were not taking anticonvulsant drugs.[7] The number of seizures increased in only eight pregnancies, and in six of these the authors thought that deprivation of sleep was important. The definition of deprivation of sleep, however, was only "a delay of more than two hours from the usual working day onset of sleep." The increase in frequency of seizures occurred most often in the first two trimesters. This proportion—one third of women having an increased frequency of seizures during pregnancy—is in accord with the wider review of Schmidt.[6] The evidence suggests that untreated epileptic pregnant women are about equally likely to experience fewer seizures during pregnancy.

Remillard et al analysed the effects of pregnancy on the different types of epileptic seizure.[8] Women with secondary generalised and complex partial seizures were most likely to have an increase in frequency of seizures during pregnancy (83% and 67% of mothers respectively). Only 29% of those with primary generalised epilepsy showed such an increase.

In a prospective study of patients receiving anticonvulsant treatment during pregnancy Schmidt et al found that the frequency of seizures increased in one third of pregnancies.[7] In two thirds of these cases the increase was associated with either poor compliance with anticonvulsant treatment or deprivation of sleep. Good compliance with anticonvulsant treatment is not easily attained. Pregnant women in developed countries are increasingly aware of the teratogenic effects of anticonvulsant drugs (see below), and they may therefore reduce or stop the prescribed regimen in an attempt to reduce the chances of having an abnormal baby.

Among pregnant epileptic women as a group, whether receiving anticonvulsant treatment or not, those who had not had a tonic-clonic seizure in the year before pregnancy, who had only one type of seizure, and who had primarily generalised epilepsy were the least likely to have an increase in frequency of seizures during pregnancy.[7] These factors are similar to those which favour good prognosis for seizures in men and non-pregnant women.[9]

Metabolism of anticonvulsant drugs during pregnancy

The writings of many authors in the United Kingdom and the United States have encouraged physicians to simplify anticonvulsant regimens to avoid adverse effects and interactions between drugs.[10] In a typical recent study nearly half of the pregnant women with epilepsy were taking only one drug.[11] The drugs most widely used are phenytoin, carbamazepine, and sodium valproate. Published work is extensive, and much of it has been collected in a monograph.[12] Only examples will be given here.

Absorption

Absorption of anticonvulsant drugs from the bowel may be reduced during pregnancy. Ramsey et al reported a pregnant woman with seizures who had low serum concentrations of phenytoin, complicated by the occurrence of status epilepticus, until the oral dosage of phenytoin was increased to 1200 mg a day.[13] Metabolic studies showed that the proportion of unmetabolised phenytoin in the urine remained unchanged but a large proportion (56%; normal range 5–15%) was excreted in the stool. This proportion fell to 23% after delivery. The malabsorption was not specific for phenytoin, also affecting xylose and dietary fat.

Distribution

During pregnancy fluid retention and the volume of fetal tissues and placenta increase the available volume for distribution of anticonvulsant drugs. This dilution tends to lower the serum concentration if the oral dose is not changed. The figure shows the fall in serum phenytoin concentration which may occur during pregnancy, although this is not due to dilutional effects alone (see below). In a recent study Jensen showed that the increase in the volume of distribution of both carbamazepine and phenytoin could not be accounted for by weight gain alone, which suggests some increased tissue affinity for these drugs during pregnancy (Jensen NO, International League against Epilepsy, York 1986).

Protein binding

Ruprah et al found that binding of phenytoin to plasma proteins was considerably reduced in the last trimester.[14] A reduction in binding changes the relation between the serum concentration of phenytoin and its therapeutic effect since a greater proportion of the drug is free and pharmacologically active. The clinical value of measuring phenytoin concentrations in whole serum is therefore greatly reduced unless serum binding is also measured. It is insufficient to judge the extent of protein binding by measuring the concentration of plasma albumin because this correlates poorly with protein binding. Direct measurement of protein binding is time consuming and requires a considerable volume of blood. Knott et al found, however, that the concentration of phenytoin in saliva measured during the pregnancies of 11 epileptic mothers correlated with the fraction of phenytoin that was unbound.[15] The correlation was sufficiently close to allow the ratio of saliva and plasma phenytoin concentration measured at the same time to be used as an index of the free fraction. The figure shows the fall in saliva phenytoin concentration during pregnancy, and hence the reduced biological effect, despite an increase in the saliva to plasma ratio, indicating reduced binding. The concentration of phenytoin can be measured in very small volumes of saliva. Some workers believe that citric acid crystals should not be used as a sialagogue if the drug is assayed by an enzyme multiplied immunoassay technique QST as the enzyme used in the assay may be inhibited by the resulting low pH.[16]

Some anticonvulsant drugs are present in fetal blood in lower concentrations than in maternal blood, but others may accumulate in the fetus so that fetal blood concentrations exceed those of the mother. Some of the difference may be accounted for by higher concentrations of drug binding proteins on one side of the placenta. Krauer measured changes in serum albumin and α_1-acid glycoprotein in paired maternal and fetal blood and showed differential changes in the ratios during pregnancy.[17] Difficulties in analysing these changes are compounded by the changes in maternal blood free fatty acids, which displace some drugs from proteins in maternal serum. Increased concentrations of drugs in fetal blood can therefore result from decreased concentrations of drug binding proteins in the mother or increased concentrations of displacing agents. The increased concentration of free fatty acids in both mother and child at birth can result in decreased protein binding of diazepam and valproic acid,[18 19] but the importance of the increased drug concentrations at this time is uncertain. Changes during early pregnancy may well be important, however, because an increase in the free fraction of anticonvulsant drugs in the fetus may lead to a greater risk of fetal abnormality. For example, Krauer et al have shown that the free fraction of diazepam in fetal serum is considerably increased in early pregnancy.[20]

Clearance

The maternal liver usually develops an increased capacity for hydroxylation of some anticonvulsant drugs such as phenytoin.[21] Lander et al found that in pregnant women the clearance of phenytoin after intravenous injection was roughly twice the rate found in non-pregnant women patients.[22] In five patients studied before and during pregnancy Jensen found increases in urinary excretion of parahydroxyphenytoin—the principal metabolite of phenytoin—ranging from 16% to 143% compared with values before pregnancy, and body clearance increased by 13% to 73% (International League against Epilepsy, York 1986). In Jensen's study the patients had been taking phenytoin for at least one year before the first estimation (while not pregnant), and so the results could not be due to the induction of hydroxylating enzymes by phenytoin itself but must represent a change associated with pregnancy. Jensen also reported increases in the clearance of carbamazepine of up to 30% in six patients and increases in the urinary excretion of trans-10,11-dihydroxycarbamazepine, the principal metabolite of carbamazepine, of 32-138%. Bardy et al, on the other hand, did not find significant changes in the clearance of carbamazepine, though the clearance of phenobarbitone was considerably increased.[23] There were striking variations within and between individuals in the clearance of primidone, but overall no significant changes were found.

The increased clearance of anticonvulsant drugs and the changes in volume of distribution may well result in a fall in serum concentration (figure). It must, however, be remembered that such a fall does not necessarily reflect changes in free concentration of anticonvulsant drugs such as phenytoin due to changes in protein

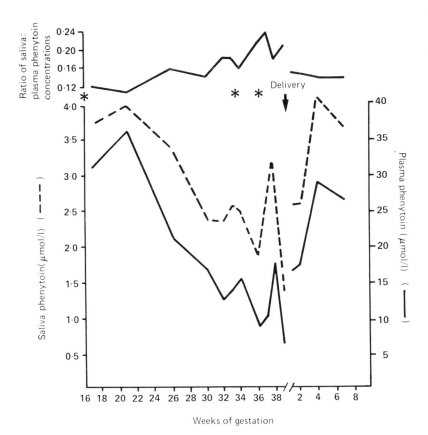

Concentrations of phenytoin in saliva and plasma and (top) ratio between the two (saliva:plasma). Although saliva and plasma concentrations roughly follow each other, there is a significant increase in ratio throughout pregnancy, reflecting increased amount of drug which is not bound to plasma protein. Probably only the unbound fraction of the drug is pharmacologically active. Asterisks indicate seizures. The break in the abscissa indicates delivery.

Data reproduced by kind permission from Knott C, Williams CP, Reynolds F. Phenytoin kinetics during pregnancy and the puerperium. *Br J Obstet Gynaecol* 1986;**93**:1030–7.

binding. Any woman with active epilepsy who becomes pregnant will therefore need regular estimations of concentrations of anticonvulsant drugs in serum and saliva with appropriate adjustment, usually an increase, of oral dosage. Close liaison between the obstetrician, neurologist, and mother is advisable. If the oral dosage of an anticonvulsant drug is increased during pregnancy appropriate adjustments must be made after delivery in order to avoid intoxication.

Drug interactions

Phenytoin interacts with many other drugs.[24] For example, benzodiazepines, which may be given to anxious pregnant women with epilepsy, lower the serum concentration of phenytoin.

Epilepsy and fetal abnormality

Effects of the seizures

Apart from the possibility of a genetic association between epilepsy and the risk of fetal abnormality (see below), seizures could cause fetal damage through hypoxia or associated trauma. Fetal monitoring during a maternal tonic-clonic seizure lasting three minutes showed that the onset of the seizure was immediately followed by fetal bradycardia lasting about 15 minutes.[25] Prolonged maternal seizures, or status epilepticus, could therefore harm the fetus. Suggested regimens for managing status epilepticus in pregnancy have been published,[26] but, with the exception of the need for fetal monitoring, they do not differ appreciably from usual medical management. In one study the highest malformation rate was for pregnancies in which seizures had occurred despite drug treatment, though the numbers were insufficient to make this association significant.[27] Although a fall during a seizure could damage the fetus, such an event must be extremely rare. There is also no evidence to suggest that obstetric complications, such as pre-eclampsia, accidental haemorrhage, or hyperemesis, are more common in epileptic mothers.[28 29]

One Scandinavian study suggested that obstetricians may be more likely to attempt potentially harmful obstetric intervention,

103

such as induction of labour and instrumental delivery, in pregnant women with epilepsy,[30] although this is seldom indicated. Another study, however, did not show an excess of such interventions.[25]

Genetic association of epilepsy and fetal abnormality

Facial clefts and cleft palate are among the most common fetal abnormalities associated with epilepsy and its treatment. The role of treatment in causing such abnormalities is considered below, although genetic factors could be responsible for both the epilepsy and the malformations. Alternatively, the increased risk of fetal abnormality may be limited to families with a genetic predisposition to malformations. A recent study from Denmark showed that epileptic men did not have more children with facial clefts than men in the general population,[32] which is in contrast to results of some earlier studies. Epileptic women, however, did have more children with facial clefts (with or without cleft palates) than women in the general population, but this increased incidence occurred only after the onset of epilepsy. Genetic factors linking epilepsy and facial clefts were largely excluded by this study. The authors concluded that epilepsy itself contributes to facial clefts in offspring; the ratio between the number of observed cases and expected cases was zero for children born before the onset of epilepsy and 2·4 for children conceived after the onset of epilepsy and where no anticonvulsant treatment had been given during the pregnancy. The ratio was 4·7 if the fetus had been exposed to anticonvulsant drugs. Although this was a large scale survey, the numbers of affected children were small, and lower confidence limits for these ratios were not given.

Effects of anticonvulsant drugs on the fetus

In 1968 Meadow reported six infants with cleft lip and palate born to mothers with epilepsy who had taken anticonvulsant drugs during pregnancy.[32] Four of the children also had cardiac lesions. All of the children had an unusual facial appearance with short neck, low hairline at the back, widely spaced eyes, and minor deformities of the pinna. This report led to a large number of publications, which have been reviewed elsewhere.[12] [27] Overall, results showed that children of epileptic mothers taking drugs have roughly twice as many malformations as children of mothers in the population as a whole. Since about 3% of all newborn babies have a significant congenital abnormality the chance of the child of a mother with epilepsy having a significant abnormality are about 6%. It is probably more encouraging to talk to the mother in terms of a 94% chance of having a normal child.

If anticonvulsant drugs are necessary in early pregnancy the smallest dose that is compatible with control of seizures should be used. Factors other than the serum concentration of unbound drug may, however, be important in teratogenesis. There is good evidence of genetic predisposition to congenital abnormalities induced by phenytoin. The most striking example is a case report of fraternal heteropaternal twins born to a mother treated with phenytoin.[33] One twin had many features of the fetal hydantoin syndrome[34] and the other none. Strickler et al found that a genetic defect in detoxification of arene oxides, intermediate metabolites of phenytoin metabolism, is correlated with major congenital defects in infants born to mothers treated with phenytoin.[35]

Troxidone, now seldom used, was found to be strongly teratogenic in one multicentre study.[27] Affected children have low set, backwards sloping ears, V shaped eyebrows, anomalies of the palate, irregular teeth, and developmental delay.[36] A fetal hydantoin (phenytoin) syndrome has also been reported,[34] the affected children suffering from craniofacial abnormalities, mental retardation, and limb defects such as digital hypoplasia. Similar dysmorphic features, however, have been seen in the children of epileptic mothers treated with other anticonvulsant drugs or not treated at all,[37] and the specificity of these "syndromes" is in doubt.[38] There is little doubt, however, that sodium valproate is particularly likely to result in neural tube defects.[39] All 10 cases reported by Lindhout and Meinardi had open defects that probably would have been detected by measuring α-fetoprotein concentration in amniotic fluid and by ultrasound scanning.[39]

There have been few reports of fetal abnormality associated with carbamazepine, but this may reflect the fact that this drug has come into extensive use only in the past 12 years or so.

Other metabolic disturbances induced by anticonvulsant drugs

Serum folate concentration

Treatment with anticonvulsant drugs may result in decreased serum folate concentrations and, occasionally, megaloblastic anaemia. Hiilesmaa et al measured serum folate concentrations in 150 pregnancies of 137 epileptic mothers who received small (about 500 µg) folic acid supplements.[40] Maternal serum folate concentrations correlated inversely with serum concentrations of phenytoin and phenobarbitone but not with those of carbamazepine. Folate values usually remained well within the normal range. There was no suggestion that a low folate concentration resulted in an increased frequency of seizures. A low dose of folate supplement therefore seems to be sufficient for pregnant women with epilepsy, despite the effect of phenytoin and phenobarbitone on folic acid.

Vitamin D metabolism

Long term treatment with phenytoin and phenobarbitone has been shown to induce clinical osteomalacia and rickets and, more commonly, hypocalcaemia without clinical evidence of bone disease. Phenobarbitone and phenytoin increase with the hepatic metabolism of vitamin D and 25-hydroxyvitamin D with depletion of vitamin stores. It has also been suggested that these drugs may modify the metabolism of dihydroxyvitamin D or inhibit intestinal absorption of minerals through mechanisms independent of any effect on vitamin D metabolism. Markestad et al showed that pregnant epileptic women who were taking anticonvulsant drugs and receiving 400 IU of vitamin D_3 a day had lower median concentrations of 25-hydroxyvitamin D and 1,25 dihydroxyvitamin D and higher median 25,26 dihydroxyvitamin D concentrations than a control group of pregnant women who also received 400 IU of vitamin D_3 each day.[41] Serum calcium concentrations tended to be lower in the women with epilepsy, but it is unlikely that these metabolic effects would be clinically important in developed countries. Asian epileptic mothers who have migrated to less sunny climates may be at risk, however, as may their babies.

Thyroid function

Although the thyroxine concentration of cord serum is significantly reduced in the infants of epileptic mothers treated with anticonvulsant drugs, this effect is entirely due to altered protein binding.[42] Phenytoin competes for thyroxine binding sites on thyroxine binding globulin.

Vitamin K metabolism

Neonates born to mothers with epilepsy who have been treated with anticonvulsant drugs are at increased risk of haemorrhage. The mechanism of this has been partly illuminated by studies on prothrombin and vitamin K. The carboxylation of an inert precursor of prothrombin in the liver is carried out by a vitamin K dependent enzyme, γ carboxylase. In the absence of vitamin K, or in the presence of vitamin K antagonists, γ carboxylase is inhibited and the inert precursor—known as protein induced by vitamin K absence (PIVKA)—appears in the serum. Davies *et al* have shown that concentrations of protein induced by vitamin K absence are raised in men and women with epilepsy treated with phenytoin, carbamazepine, sodium valproate, and phenobarbitone without any biochemical evidence of hepatic dysfunction.[43] Neonatal haemorrhage can be prevented by giving women vitamin K during pregnancy.[44]

Neonatal period

The rate of clearance of anticonvulsant drugs from newborn babies has been reviewed by Bossi.[45] The half life of sodium valproate is 14–88 hours, primidone 7–60 hours, phenobarbitone 40-500 hours, phenytoin 15–105 hours, and carbamazepine 8–28 hours.

The clinical signs of barbiturate withdrawal in the neonate are hyperexcitability, occasional seizures, tremulousness, and impaired suckling.[46] Kaneko *et al* found less efficient suckling and slower weight gain in the infants of epileptic mothers than in the infants of normal mothers.[47] Expectant supervision of such children is usually adequate, but if tremulousness or, in particular, seizures occur, small doses of phenobarbitone (3–5 mg/kg/day) may be given.

Breast feeding

Most mothers taking anticonvulsant drugs may safely breast feed their children. Significant amounts of these drugs do, however, pass into the milk.[47 48] The ratio between the concentration in breast milk and serum concentration is 0·19 for phenytoin, 0·41 for carbamazepine, 0·36 for phenobarbitone, and 0·70 for primidone.[47] In practice, phenytoin and carbamazepine have little clinical effect on the neonate.

Conclusions

An epileptic woman of childbearing age who has had no seizures for two or three years should have anticonvulsant treatment gradually withdrawn before any planned pregnancy. For a woman who needs anticonvulsant drugs the dose should be as low as possible. Serum or saliva concentrations of anticonvulsant drugs should be monitored during pregnancy because there are considerable changes in pharmacokinetics. There is a risk of teratogenesis; the risk seems to be least for carbamazepine. Readjustment of dosage is necessary in the puerperium. Mothers taking anticonvulsant drugs may safely breast feed their children.

Some of this chapter is based on material that appeared in de Swiet M, ed. *Medical Disorders in Obstetric Practice*. Oxford: Blackwell Scientific, 1984.

1 Hauser WA, Kurland LT. The epidemiology of epilepsy in Rochester, Minnesota, 1935 through 1967. *Epilepsia* 1975;**16**:1–66.
2 Knight AH, Rhind EG. Epilepsy and pregnancy: a study of 153 pregnancies in 59 patients. *Epilepsia* 1975;**16**:99–110.
3 Haas JF, Janisch W, Staneczek W. Newly diagnosed primary intracranial neoplasms in pregnant women: a population-based assessment. *J Neurol Neurosurg Psychiatry* 1986;**49**:874–80.
4 Bickerstaff ER, Small JM, Guest LA. The relapsing course of certain meningiomas in relation to pregnancy and menstruation *J Neurol Neurosurg Psychiatry* 1958;**21**:89–94.
5 Kalbag RM, Woolf AL. *Cerebral venous thrombosis*. Oxford: Oxford University Press, 1967.
6 Schmidt D. The effect of pregnancy on the natural history of epilepsy: review of the literature. In: Janz D, Dam M, Richens A, Bossi L, Helge H, Schmidt D, eds. *Epilepsy, pregnancy and the child*. New York: Raven Press, 1982:3–14.
7 Schmidt D, Canger R, Avanzini G, et al. Change of seizure frequency in pregnant epileptic women. *J Neurol Neurosurg Psychiatry* 1983;**46**:751–5.

8 Remillard G, Dansky L, Andermann E, Andermann F. Seizure frequency during pregnancy and the puerperium. In: Janz D, Dam M, Richens A, Bossi L, Helge H, Schmidt D, eds. *Epilepsy, pregnancy and the child.* New York: Raven Press, 1982:15–26.

9 Rodin E. *The prognosis of patients with epilepsy.* Springfield: C Thomas, 1968.

10 Porter RJ. *Epilepsy: 100 elementary principles.* London: WB Saunders, 1984.

11 Kallen, B. A register study of maternal epilepsy and delivery outcome with special reference to drug use. *Acta Neurol Scand* 1986;**73**:253–9.

12 Janz D, Dam M, Richens A, Bossi L, Helge H, Schmidt D. *Epilepsy, pregnancy and the child.* New York: Raven Press, 1982.

13 Ramsey RE, Strauss RG, Willmore LJ. Status epilepticus in pregnancy: effects of phenytoin malabsorption on seizure control. *Neurology* 1978;**28**:85–9.

14 Ruprah M, Perucca E, Richens A. Decreased serum protein binding of phenytoin in late pregnancy. *Lancet* 1980;ii:316–7.

15 Knott C, Williams CP, Reynolds F. Phenytoin kinetics during pregnancy and the puerperium. *Br J Obstet Gynaecol* 1986;**93**:1030–7.

16 Paton RD, Logan RW. Salivary drug measurement: a cautionary tale. *Lancet* 1986;ii:1340.

17 Krauer B, Dayer P, Anner R. Changes in serum albumin and 1-acid glycoprotein concentrations during pregnancy: an analysis of fetal-maternal pairs. *Br J Obstet Gynaecol* 1984;**91**:875–81.

18 Nau H, Luck W, Kuhnz W. Decreased serum protein binding of diazepam and its major metabolite in the neonate during the first post-natal week relate to increased free fatty acid levels. *Br J Clin Pharmacol* 1984;**17**:92–8.

19 Nau H, Helge H, Luck W. Valproic acid in the perinatal period: decreased maternal serum protein binding results in fetal accumulation and neonatal displacement of the drug and some metabolites. *J Pediatr* 1984;**104**:627–34.

20 Krauer B, Nau H, Dayer P, Bischoff P, Anner R. Serum protein binding of diazepam and propranolol in the feto-maternal unit from early to late pregnancy. *Br J Obstet Gynaecol* 1986;**93**:322–8.

21 Mygind KI, Dam M, Christiansen J. Phenytoin and phenobarbitone plasma clearance during pregnancy. *Acta Neurol Scand* 1976;**54**:160–6.

22 Lander CM, Smith MT, Chalk JB, et al. Bioavailability and pharmacokinetics of phenytoin during pregnancy. *Eur J Clin Pharmacol* 1984;**27**:105–10.

23 Bardy AH, Teramo K, Hiilesmaa VK. Apparent plasma clearances of phenytoin, phenobarbitone, primidone and carbamazepine during pregnancy: results of the prospective Helsinki study. In: Janz D, Dam M, Richens A, Bossi L, Helge H, Schmidt D, eds. *Epilepsy, pregnancy and the child.* New York: Raven Press, 1982:141–5.

24 Richens A. *Drug treatment of epilepsy.* London: Henry Kimpton, 1976.

25 Hiilesmaa VK, Bardy A, Terano R. Obstetric outcome in women with epilepsy. *Am J Obstet Gynecol* 1985;**152**:499–504.

26 Dalessio DJ. Seizure disorders and pregnancy. *N Engl J Med* 1985;**312**:559–63.

27 Nakane Y, Okuma T, Takahishi R, et al. Multi-institutional study on the teratogenecity and fetal toxicity of anti-epileptic drugs: a report of a collaboration study group in Japan. *Epilepsia* 1980;**21**:663–80.

28 Philbert A, Dam M. The epileptic mother and her child. *Epilepsia* 1982;**23**:85–99.

29 Yerby M, Koepsell T, Daling D. Pregnancy complications and outcome in a cohort of women with epilepsy. *Epilepsia* 1985;**26**:631–5.

30 Egenaes J. Outcome of pregnancy in women with epilepsy, Norway 1967–1978: description of material. In: Janz D, Dam M, Richens A, Bossi L, Helge H, Schmidt D, eds. *Epilepsy, pregnancy and the child.* New York: Raven Press, 1982:81–5.

31 Friis ML, Holm NV, Sindrup EH, Fogh-Andersen P, Hauge M. Facial clefts in sibs and children of epileptic patients. *Neurology* 1986;**36**:346–50.

32 Meadow SR. Anticonvulsant drugs and congenital abnormalities. *Lancet* 1968;ii:1296.

33 Phelan MC, Pellock JM, Nance WE. Discordant expresson of fetal hydantoin syndrome in heteropaternal dizygotic twins. *N Engl J Med* 1982;**307**:99–102.

34 Hanson JW, Smith DW. The fetal hydantoin syndrom. *J Pediatr* 1975;**87**:285–90.

35 Strickler SM, Miller MA, Andermann E. Genetic predisposition to phenytoin-induced birth defects. *Lancet* 1985;ii:746–9.

36 Zackai EH, Mellman WJ, Neiderer B, Hanson JW. The fetal trimethadione syndrome. *J Pediatr* 1975;**87**:285–90.

37 Meadow SR. The teratogenic asociation of epilepsy and anticonvulsant drugs. In: Hopkins A, ed. *Epilepsy*. London: Chapman and Hall (in press).

38 Livingston J, Lyall H. Contribution of fetal alcohol syndrome to mental retardation: *Lancet* 1986;ii:1337–8.

39 Lindhout D, Meinardi H. Spina bifida and in-utero exposure to valproate. *Lancet* 1984;ii:396.

40 Hiilesmaa VE, Teramo K, Granstrom M-L, Bardy AH. Serum folate concentrations in women with epilepsy. *Br Med J* 1983;285:577–9.

41 Markestad T, Ulstein M, Strandjord RE, Akanes L, Arskog D. Anticonvulsant drug therapy in human pregnancy: effects on serum concentrations of vitamin D metabolites in maternal and cord blood. *Am J Obstet Gynecol* 1984;150:254–8.

42 Carriero R, Andermann E, Moy-Fung Chen MD, *et al.* Thyroid function in epileptic mothers and their infants at birth. *Am J Obstet Gynecol* 1985;151:641–4.

43 Davies VA, Argent AC, Staub H, *et al.* Precursor prothrombin status in patients receiving anticonvulsant drugs. *Lancet* 1985;i:126–8.

44 Deblay MF. Vert P, Andre M, Marchal F. Transplacental vitamin K prevents haemorrhagic disease of infant of epileptic mother. *Lancet* 1982;i:1247.

45 Bossi L. Neonatal period including drug disposition in newborns: review of the literature. In: Janz D, Dam M, Richens A, Bossi L, Helge H, Schmidt D, eds. *Epilepsy, pregnancy and the child*. New York: Raven Press, 1982:327–34.

46 Desmond MM, Schwanecke RP, Wilson GS, *et al.* Maternal barbiturate utilisation and neonatal withdrawal symptomatology. *J Pediatr* 1972;80:190–7.

47 Kaneko S, Suzuki K, Sato T, Ogawa Y, Nomura Y. The problems of antiepileptic medication in the neonatal period: is breast feeding advisable? In: Janz D, Dam M, Richens A, Bossi L, Helge H, Schmidt D, eds. *Epilepsy, pregnancy and the child*. New York: Raven Press 1982:343–8.

48 Nau H, Cuhnz W, Egger HJ, Rating D, Helge H. Anticonvulsants during pregnancy and lactation. *Clin Pharmacokinet* 1982;7:508–43.

Treatment of diabetes

N J A VAUGHAN

The importance of a good metabolic control in pregnant women with diabetes is now undisputed. Complications such as macrosomia, neonatal hypoglycaemia, intrauterine death, and hydramnios can largely be prevented by intensive efforts to achieve strict normoglycaemia, and many centres now report perinatal mortality in the babies of women with insulin dependent diabetes approaching the rate found in the general population—that is, 1·6–2%. The use of home blood glucose monitoring, education about diabetes, and outpatient methods of fetal surveillance have been central to this improvement. Great emphasis is placed on team care, the team comprising diabetologist, obstetrician, diabetic nurse, paediatrician, and, most importantly, the patient. As a consequence, admission to hospital has been minimised, and there is a well established trend towards allowing uncomplicated pregnancies in diabetic women to go to term.

Perhaps the most important decision is the choice of insulin treatment both before and during pregnancy. Insulin treatment must be tailored to the individual. Each patient should have an insulin regimen which provides a degree of flexibility that enables a normal blood glucose concentration (3–6 mmol/l (54–108 mg/ml)) to be maintained throughout the day and night and which will also accommodate increasing insulin requirements as gestation progresses. This chapter outlines the available options of insulin treatment both for women with insulin dependent diabetes diagnosed before the onset of pregnancy and for those with gestational diabetes requiring insulin treatment. The question of whether insulin should be given in cases of gestational diabetes is not discussed as this is well reviewed elsewhere.[1-3]

Prepregnancy counselling

Pregnancies in diabetic women should be planned. All insulin dependent women of childbearing age who envisage pregnancy should be advised of the need for good control well before any attempts to conceive. Despite the dramatic reductions in many of the complications, the incidence of congenital anomalies in children of diabetic mothers remains three times greater than the incidence in the general population, and fatal anomalies and multiple malformations still occur six times as often. Organogenesis for all sites in which the congenital anomalies of children with diabetic mothers are most common is essentially complete within the first six weeks of gestation—that is before the mother may know she is pregnant.

Pregnancy should ideally be deferred until prolonged good metabolic control has been attained. Suitable evidence of this would be glycosylated haemoglobin values at or below the upper limit of normal. To achieve good metabolic control it is probably simplest if the insulin regimen that is planned for the pregnancy is started in this preconception period. All women who could possibly become pregnant should now be using human insulin. Patients who are still using porcine or, especially, bovine insulin preparations should be changed to the corresponding human formulations and their regimen optimised.

Dietary prescription in pregnant women with diabetes

An adequate diet is essential in the management of pregnancy in a diabetic woman. It has to meet the nutritional needs of both mother and fetus and provide a total daily energy requirement during pregnancy of 35–38 kcal/kg non-pregnant ideal body weight. Fewer calories than this will not allow efficient protein utilisation and may lead to ketogenesis induced by starvation. It is recommended that not less than 200 g carbohydrate daily is consumed and that this should comprise at least 45% of the total daily calorie intake. This carbohydrate should be distributed throughout the day as regular meals and snacks, and it is especially important to provide a substantial bedtime snack (25 g carbohydrate and some protein). This helps to prevent starvation ketosis in the morning and to avoid nocturnal hypoglycaemia. High dietary fibre content may improve metabolic control. This may be achieved by dietary manipulation[4] or by the addition of gel forming supplements such as guar gum.[5] Protein requirements increase by about 30 g a day during pregnancy, and an intake of 1·3 g/kg body weight will generally meet maternal and fetal needs, although pregnant adolescents may require more (1·5–1·7 g/kg).

There is little or no place for calorie restriction in the control of diabetes in pregnancy. Nevertheless, in mild gestational diabetes it is usually worth attempting to correct a previously poor eating pattern. Good metabolic control can occasionally be achieved by dietary measures, but such patients must be watched carefully with frequent checks on blood glucose and glycosylated haemoglobin values. Any suspicion of deteriorating control requires the immediate introduction of insulin.

Insulin treatment

Several factors must be taken into account when selecting an insulin regimen. Nothing less than the attainment of normal blood glucose values throughout the day and night should be acceptable to either the patient or her physician. Regular home blood glucose measurements, preferably with a reflectance meter, are essential, not only to meet day to day variations in blood glucose concentration but also to keep up with increasing insulin requirements as pregnancy progresses. Given this degree of documentation, along with the patient's almost invariably higher motivation and the fact that the metabolic changes of pregnancy generally make diabetes easier to control, it is possible to achieve sufficiently good control with most insulin regimens that entail two or more injections of a mixture of insulins. Although not always practicable, it is probably best if radical changes in strategy are avoided and that any changes are made gradually as pregnancy progresses.

Choice of insulin species

With the ready availability of human insulin in most formulations the question of insulin species will soon cease to be an issue. Most patients, however, use highly purified porcine or bovine insulins. Insulin antibodies, which may be produced in mothers treated with insulin, can freely cross the placenta.[6] They have been implicated as a cause of infant morbidity, possibly affecting β-cell function of the fetus and influencing neonatal insulin secretion.[7 8] It is therefore logical to treat pregnant women with insulin formulations of minimum antigenicity. Single peak insulins contain contaminants that render them sufficiently antigenic to exclude their use in pregnancy. Bovine insulins, which are inherently more antigenic than porcine or human preparations, should also not be used. Human insulin is less antigenic than porcine insulin, although the differences are small. Thus patients who have not previously received insulin should be given human insulin. Intermittent exposure to an antigen encourages antibody formation, and this is an important consideration when using insulin in gestational diabetes. As previously indicated, a change to human insulin preparations in insulin dependent diabetics is best performed before conception.

Choice of insulin regimens

Once daily insulin—Although seldom appropriate in pregnant women with diabetes, single daily injections of an intermediate duration insulin before breakfast, sometimes in combination with a short acting insulin, may be effective in some women with mild gestational diabetes.[9 10] Such diabetics can usually produce sufficient insulin to keep blood glucose concentrations normal in the fasting state and therefore require insulin cover for only about 15 hours a day. This can be provided by a human insulin zinc suspension: Human Monotard (Novo) or Humulin Zn (Lilly). Alternatively, a human isophane insulin—Protophane (Novo), Humulin I (Lilly), or Human Insulatard (Nordisk)—may be used. Additional Human Actrapid (Novo) or Humulin S (Lilly) provides a fast acting component to prevent postprandial hyperglycaemia during the morning. The use of such regimens significantly reduces the incidence of fetal macrosomia in women with mild gestational diabetes when compared with treatment by diet alone.[10]

Short and intermediate insulin combinations twice daily—This regimen is widely used outside pregnancy and often provides adequate control during pregnancy. The usual combinations are a soluble insulin with either an isophane insulin or an insulin zinc suspension such as Monotard. Although premixed formulations of soluble and isophane insulins are now available, to retain maximal flexibility in pregnancy it is preferable to draw these insulins up in tailor made proportions. Humulin S and Humulin I, Human Actrapid and Protophane, or Human Velosulin and Human Insulatard are all suitable combinations. Tailor made mixtures are particularly useful because as pregnancy progresses the required balance between short and intermediate action may change by virtue of increasing insulin resistance and also an increasing rate of transfer of glucose to the fetus.

A general guide for the initial distribution of insulin is to give two thirds of the total daily dose in the morning and one third in the evening. Usually, 30% soluble and 70% isophane insulin will suit early pregnancy, but as gestation progresses the proportion of isophane insulin required in the morning may fall, reflecting increased insulin resistance. Equally, the evening doses of isophane insulin may also have to be reduced to avoid hypoglycaemia during the latter part of the night as a result of increased transplacental passage of glucose. These proportions must be selected on the basis of home blood glucose estimations before meals and bedtime. The importance of a mid-morning snack must be emphasised if hypoglycaemia before lunch is to be avoided. In the case of hyperglycaemia before breakfast an increased evening dose of isophane insulin may not be sufficient to overcome this without causing nocturnal hypoglycaemia. A solution to this is to split the evening combination of insulins, moving the isophane injection to bedtime.

Multiple daily insulin injections—It is sometimes both easier and more satisfactory to use numerous small injections of a short acting insulin related to food intake with a single daily dose of a long acting insulin. Most effective is the use of Humulin S, Human Actrapid, or Human Velosulin at breakfast, lunch, and supper with a human isophane insulin or Human Ultratard at bedtime. This type of regimen is readily understood by the patient and can easily be varied from day to day to cope with varying activity or diet. Furthermore, the various pen injectors that are now appearing designed specifically for such regimens are making multiple injection much more acceptable. The most familiar variety at the moment is probably the Novopen, although another type, Insuject (Nordisk), will soon be available. Novopen takes Penfill cartridges that contain 150 units of Human Actrapid, usually enough to last

Treatment of diabetic ketoacidosis

Pregnant women with diabetes are much more prone to diabetic ketoacidosis than other diabetics because of the combination of insulin resistance and accelerated catabolism in pregnancy. Initiating factors are the same as for any diabetic and include vomiting, infections, failure of insulin administration, or failure to meet increasing insulin requirements.

Ketoacidosis in pregnancy must be treated with the utmost urgency as fetal loss occurs in almost half of all cases. Patients should be managed on a medical intensive care unit along conventional lines. Adequate fluid and potassium replacement is required in conjunction with intravenous insulin infusion adjusted to achieve a smooth reduction of plasma glucose concentration to normal. Initial rehydration should be with normal saline; this should be changed to dextrose once the blood glucose concentration is less than 10 mmol/l (180 mg/100 ml) and continued until the patient is free of ketones.

The use of corticosteroids in premature labour before 34 weeks' gestation to accelerate fetal lung maturation may dramatically increase insulin resistance. Similarly, the use of intravenous β sympathomimetic agents to treat premature uterine contractions will cause severe hyperglycaemia and ketoacidosis unless appropriately anticipated. Careful glucose monitoring should always accompany this form of treatment and aggressive intravenous insulin treatment must be started if necessary.

Conclusions

Remarkable improvements in the prognosis for diabetic pregnancy have been achieved in the past two decades. Consensus now dictates that efforts to achieve strict control should be directed not only at pregnancy itself but also at the preconception period. For a successful outcome close cooperation is required between physician, obstetrician, paediatrician, and patient. Appropriate nutritional advice is an important aspect of management that should not be forgotten. Choice of insulin regimens may at first appear bewilderingly diverse, but whether this entails two, three, or four injections a day is important only in so far as it meets the patient's individual requirements to achieve normoglycaemia. No individual regimen can be claimed to be ideal; much depends on the patient's cooperation and understanding. Complex regimens are not a substitute for diabetic education and careful monitoring.

1 O'Sullivan JB. Establishing criteria for gestational diabetes. *Diabetes Care* 1980;3:437–9.
2 Gabbe SG. Effects of identifying a high risk population. *Diabetes Care* 1980;3:486–8.
3. Friend JR. Diabetes. *Clin Obstet Gynaecol* 1981;8:353–82.
4 Ney D, Hollingworth DR, Cousins L. Decreased insulin requirements and improved control of diabetes in pregnant women given a high in carbohydrate, high fibre, low fat diet. *Diabetes Care* 1982;5:529–33.
5 Gabbe SG, Cohen AW, Herman GO, Schwartz S. Effect of dietary fibre on the oral glucose tolerance test in pregnancy. *Am J Obstet Gynecol* 1982;143:514–7.
6 Bauman WA, Yalow RS. Placental passage of antibody and insulin-antibody complexes. *Diabetes* 1982;31:suppl 2: 154A, 589.
7 Heding LG, Persson B, Strangenburg M. B-cell function in newborn infants of diabetic mothers. *Diabetologia* 1980;19:427–32.
8 Persson B, Heding LG, Lunell NO, *et al*. Fetal B-cell function in diabetic pregnancy, amniotic fluid concentrations of proinsulin, insulin and C-peptide during the last trimester of pregnancy. *Am J Obstet Gynecol* 1982;144:455–9.
9 O'Sullivan JB, Mahan CM, Charles D, Dandrow RV. Medical treatment of the gestational diabetic. *Obstet Gynecol* 1974;43:817–21.
10 Coustan DR, Lewis SB. Insulin therapy for gestational diabetes. *Obstet Gynecol* 1978;51:306–10.
11 Pickup JC, Keen H, Parsons JA, Alberti KGMM. Continuous subcutaneous insulin infusion: an approach to achieving normoglycaemia. *Br Med J* 1978;i:204–7.
12 Rizza RA, Gerich JE, Haymond MW, *et al*. Control of blood sugar in insulin dependent diabetes: comparison of an artificial endocrine pancreas, continuous subcutaneous insulin infusion and intensified conventional therapy. *N Engl J Med* 1980;303:1313–8.
13 Reeves M, Siegler D, Ryan E, Skyler J. Glycemic control in insulin dependent diabetes mellitus—a comparison of outpatient intensified conventional therapy with continuous subcutaneous insulin infusion. *Am J Med* 1982;72:673–80.
14 Roversi GD, Gargiulo M, Nicolini U, *et al*. Maximal tolerated insulin therapy in gestational diabetes. *Diabetes Care* 1980;3:489–94.
15 Adam PAJ, Schwartz R. Diagnosis and treatment: should oral hypoglycaemic agents be used in paediatric and pregnant patients. *Paediatrics* 1968;42:819–23.
16 Sutherland HW, Stowers JM, Cormack JD, Bewsher PD. Evaluation of chlorpropamide in chemical diabetes diagnosed during pregnancy. *Br Med J* 1973;ii:9–13.
17 Coetzee EJ, Jackson WP. Metformin in the management of pregnant non-insulin dependent diabetes. *Diabetologia* 1979;16: 241–5.
18 Feeney JG. Water intoxication and oxytocin. *Br Med J* 1982;285:243.